"*Eat Naked* is full of convincing argume
the junk out of your diet and replaci
exactly what needs to happen."

—Mark Bittman, columnist for the *New York Times* and author
of *How to Cook Everything* and *The Food Matters Cookbook*

"Eating naked is not The Next Diet. It is The Last Diet. Purge your
pantry and strip the junk from your shopping list, but beware: you will
doubtless have to face the facts about your rotten little food habits.
Mine was surimi."

—Nina Planck, author of *Real Food: What to Eat and Why*

"Margaret Floyd's *Eat Naked* is a clear and passionate call to nourish
ourselves in a more simple, natural, and beautiful way. With just the
right mixture of science and sass, *Eat Naked* delivers wise nutritional
information that's easy to practice. In a world overloaded with conflict-
ing dietary facts and systems, Margaret Floyd gracefully distills some of
the best strategies for vibrant eating and living."

—Marc David, author of *The Slow Down Diet* and founder of
the Institute for the Psychology of Eating

"*Eat Naked* is wildly intriguing. For all time, our ancestors ate food that
was caught wild, grass-fed, fermented, unprocessed, whole, and natural.
In the last hundred years, these necessary, nourishing human traditions
have been lost, and we're largely at the mercy of Big Agriculture and
the food industry. *Eat Naked* is a food revolution book that sets you
free and also sets you on fire—free to live a long, fertile, healthy life of
personal responsibility without disease, and on fire, because real access
to whole foods is the newest civil rights movement that affects us all.
Eat naked and thrive!"

—Mark McAfee, founder of Organic Pastures Dairy

"In *Eat Naked*, Margaret Floyd has created an easy-to-follow guide to
optimizing your health. Drawing on basic principles, Floyd teaches her
readers how to cook and eat for health, healing, weight loss, and for the
pure love of food. Everyone should eat naked."

—Joshua Rosenthal, founder and director of Integrative
Nutrition

"This is a user-friendly, well-written book with sound and sensible nutritional information. The recipes are good, and easy, too!"

—Annemarie Colbin, PhD, founder and CEO of the National Gourmet Institute in New York, NY, and author of *Food and Healing* and *The Whole-Food Guide to Strong Bones*

"Empowering, and simplified to a doable matrix, *Eat Naked* gets rid of the fluff and complexity surrounding locally sourced, home-prepared eating and puts it within reach of anyone. What a wonderful contribution to this movement."

—Joel Salatin, co-owner of Polyface Farm

"As a certified personal trainer, I thought I was eating a very healthy diet. When I worked with Margaret, I realized that I was not getting the proper nutrition that my body needed. Sometimes I can't believe that I can really eat butter and not feel guilty! I can't believe that after years of dieting, my weight has stabilized and I never feel deprived."

—Christi Schimpke, CPT, National Academy of Sports Medicine, client

"This amazing eating philosophy has yielded two unexpected and surprising results. First, I'm enjoying eating more than ever before while eating foods I love, like avocados and bacon. Second, as I have learned to relate to food differently and be mindful about what I eat and how I eat, my body image has seemingly magically improved. Eating naked is so much more than a nutritional program. It's a new way to think about food and pleasure, life and self."

—Michael Douglas, client

"Eating naked has transformed my life completely, allowing me to lose unwanted weight and feel healthier and more powerful every day of my life. The increased energy I have supports my career and relationship growth, empowering me to live my dreams. For me, eating naked has become a way of life, the naked life!"

—April Kuramoto, client, yoga instructor, and BLYS Yoga Studio founder and owner

eat ™
naked
margaret floyd

**UNPROCESSED, UNPOLLUTED, and UNDRESSED
EATING for a HEALTHIER, SEXIER YOU**

New Harbinger Publications, Inc.

Publisher's Note

This publication is designed to provide accurate and authoritative information in regard to the subject matter covered. It is sold with the understanding that the publisher is not engaged in rendering psychological, financial, legal, or other professional services. If expert assistance or counseling is needed, the services of a competent professional should be sought.

Distributed in Canada by Raincoast Books

Copyright © 2011 by Margaret Floyd
        New Harbinger Publications, Inc.
        5674 Shattuck Avenue
        Oakland, CA 94609
        www.newharbinger.com

Eat Naked® is a Registered Trademark of Eat Naked, LLC, All Rights Reserved.

Cover design by Amy Shoup; Text design by Michele Waters-Kermes; Acquired by Catharine Meyers; Edited by Carole Honeychurch; Recipes co-authored by James Barry

Library of Congress Cataloging in Publication Data

Floyd, Margaret.
  Eat naked : unprocessed, unpolluted, and undressed eating for a healthier, sexier you / Margaret Floyd.
     p. cm.
  Includes bibliographical references.
  ISBN 978-1-60882-013-9 (pbk.) -- ISBN 978-1-60882-014-6 (pdf ebook) 1. Natural foods. 2. Nutrition. 3. Health. I. Title.
  TX369.F56 2011
  641.3'02--dc22

                           2011005999

FSC

Mixed Sources
Product group from well-managed forests and other controlled sources
Cert no. SW-COC-002283
www.fsc.org
© 1996 Forest Stewardship Council

13   12   11

10   9   8   7   6   5   4   3   2   1

First printing

For Gramma.
You were right. Butter is better.

Contents

Part 2: How to Get Naked

acknowledgments

The journey of writing this book has been an absolutely magical experience, and I could never have done it without the help, love, cheerleading, and endless support of some really incredible people. Starting from the beginning...

Great thanks go out to my parents, Rowland and Cynthia Floyd, for riding the often-wild waves as I stumbled along my path. You've stood by me as I took many side routes and made many a course correction to get to where I am now. You have always believed in me, you taught me what is truly important, and you have been incredibly patient and supportive of even my wildest dreams. And let us not forget the frequent-flyer points that came to my rescue and afforded me the time and space to escape my daily routine and, ultimately, come up with the idea for this book. Thank you.

I'll always be indebted to my two most formative influences in the early days, my grandmother, Margaret Millman, and my nanny, Aileen Sykes. These two incredible women were the first to introduce me to the wonders of a home-cooked meal. For that, I am forever grateful.

Thank you Mona, Shaun, and Ruby Leonard, for opening your home and kitchen to me twice for extended periods of time. It is thanks to your generosity that I was afforded the peace and quiet for the inspiration to write this book. Thank you for providing such a beautiful, comfy, and perfect space for me and my process. A big thanks to Sven Kamm, for being a key part of the early brainstorming, for encouraging me through my dark moments when it all felt impossible, and for providing such a safe space for me to write and focus on my work.

Thanks to Stephanie Losee, who made some very helpful phone calls and introduced me to Loretta Barrett, literary agent and strategic advisor extraordinaire. Loretta, navigating through this process would have been impossible without you. My two researchers, Erica Lyons and Eric Cassils, were indispensable. And my fearless reviewers, Stephanie Shearer, Dave Waite, and Debra Joy, provided such helpful input, comments, and cheerleading. They are a big part of the reason this book makes any sense at all.

I will always be indebted to the incredible chef James Barry, who is largely responsible for the tastiness, accuracy, and innovative tips included in chapter 13, "Cook Naked." It is thanks to you that the chicken stock will taste like stock and not simply warm flavored water. Jamie, I continue to learn so much from you. Your feedback, input, and strong support have been invaluable. Thank you for everything.

Many friends and colleagues provided an ear, a meal, a couch, or a pep talk. There are so many of you to name, and at risk of missing some, I'm going to try. Mellissa: for your wise words when I needed them most. Meg: for believing in me when I wasn't ready to believe in myself. Helen and Jason: for your hospitality while I madly finished up the last chapters. Laura: for your ability to pick me up, no matter how far down I'd dug my hole. Cameron: for the endless and much needed cheerleading and encouragement. Ariel: for your wisdom and ability to calm me. Leslie: for your insights and contagious laugh. Tessa: for your truth-telling and tough love when I needed it most. Deb: for your ability to see the bigger picture, always, and remind me of what's truly important.

A big shout-out to Wendy Millstine, Catharine Sutker, Jess Beebe, and the whole fabulous team at New Harbinger. Thank you for taking the risk on me and *Eat Naked*. I am honored and delighted to be publishing with you. And of course Carole Honeychurch, my incredible editor: thank you so much for the clarity and guidance you brought through this process.

And of course a huge thank you to my clients. You are my best teachers, and this book is really because of and for you.

introduction

I am absolutely thrilled to welcome you to *Eat Naked*, a whole-foods way of eating and living. This book has been a true labor of love. You hold in your hands the genesis of years of learning, reading, seeking, and teaching about nutrition, cooking, and health.

This book is for anyone who loves food, wants to eat well, wants to feel well, and doesn't want to spend loads of time trying to accomplish these things. This book is for you if you:

- Love to eat

- Want to lose some weight but don't want to diet to do so

- Want to eat healthfully without feeling deprived

- Are unwell and want to build a platform for health by giving your body what it needs to heal

- Are already quite healthy and want to maintain or even increase your health and truly thrive

- Want to learn how to prepare nutritious food in a healthful way that is simple, fast, and delicious

- Want simple guidelines on how to choose the most nutritious foods

No matter your dietary preference—vegetarian or omnivore, raw or cooked, macrobiotic, traditional, or modern—eating naked will only enhance the health benefits, simplify the process, and help you look great, even without your clothes on!

My Story

I love food. I love everything about it: growing it, cooking it, sharing it, and, most importantly, eating it. While I've always loved food, I haven't always loved healthy food, mostly because I didn't understand it and didn't really know what it was.

In the late 1990s I had my first profound experience with the power of eating naked foods when I visited a naturopath (a health care provider who uses a combination of diet, exercise, lifestyle changes, and natural therapies to improve health and treat disease). I needed to address a skin condition I'd been struggling with since my teens, and conventional Western medicine hadn't come up with a solution. At the time, I thought I already ate really well. I was a vegetarian after all, and wasn't meat the culprit of all dietary, environmental, and health woes? Looking back, I realize that I was what I now call a "junk-food vegetarian." Sure, I wasn't eating meat, but I wasn't eating healthfully either.

With an overhaul of my food—moving from a diet that included an abundance of overprocessed and refined foods to one that focused on nutrient-dense, whole or "naked" foods—I eliminated the chronic and extensive skin condition I'd suffered from for years.

From that time on, I spent the better part of my adult life in perpetual pursuit of the perfect, healthy way to eat. I looked at vegetarian and vegan diets, macrobiotic diets, traditional diets, diets based on physical characteristics like blood type, protein-based diets, low-fat diets, raw-food diets, and diets for specific health conditions. The list was nearly endless. Each diet claimed to be "the" diet that worked. And for some people, any given diet did work. But for others, it didn't.

Feeling confused, I decided to study nutrition formally, which is where I learned about the important concept of *bio-individuality*. As the saying goes, "One man's food is another man's poison." We are all unique, and a diet that works for one person doesn't necessarily work for everyone.

That said, there were some common and simple themes among the most successful diets. These commonalities weren't about calorie counting, they weren't about being vegetarian or not, and they weren't about specific ratios of protein to fat to carbohydrates. The diets that actually worked were the ones that make the most intuitive sense, that provide the most nourishing and nutrient-dense foods, that don't require deprivation, and that bring us back to real, whole foods. In other words, naked diets.

What's in This Book

This book is divided into two parts. In the first, "The Basics of Eating Naked," I explain, well, the basics. In this initial part if the book, we'll look at the principles of eating naked and then apply those principles to the basic food groups we deal with on a daily basis. What is naked meat? Is there such a thing? How do you know it's naked? What's a naked beverage? How do you find naked produce? And so on. We'll also look at why it's so important to eat naked and how non-naked foods are responsible for damaging our health and expanding our waistlines.

In "How to Get Naked," the second part of *Eat Naked*, I'll give you all the tools you'll need to begin eating naked in your own life. We're all human, and real change doesn't happen overnight. When we make quick changes, they're usually hard to sustain over time. This is one of the reasons most diets don't ultimately work. Eating naked is a lifestyle, not a diet. This is for the long term.

In part 2, I'll take you through a step-by-step process to move your diet from what it is now to a naked diet. We'll also look at techniques for finding naked food (chapter 12, "Shop Naked") and preparing naked food (chapter 13, "Cook Naked"), along with a few naked recipes to get you started. I've also included a "reality-check" chapter (chapter 15, "When *Not* to Eat Naked"), because, let's face it, sometimes a good old-fashioned hamburger from the burger joint down the street is the only thing that's going to cut it. For this to be truly sustainable and realistic for you, we've got to build in room for those moments.

What's Not in This Book

I want to take a moment to address what *isn't* in this book, because there are so many things I could have done but didn't. These omissions were quite intentional.

For one, this book is not intended to provide an in-depth look at the ins and outs of a whole-foods diet. There are some fabulous resources out there that do this brilliantly (two of my favorites are Nina Planck's 2006 *Real Food* and Sally Fallon's *Nourishing Traditions* from 2001). For another, this book is not intended to give a long history of how we got to this point in our food supply. Again, there are excellent resources that document this, Michael Pollan's *In Defense of Food* (2009) being my personal favorite.

Another thing I've not done in this book is dissect food down into its nutritional bits and pieces, nor have I focused heavily on a specific nutrient. Yes, it's important to get enough of the various macro- and micronutrients, and the individual benefits of some of these are truly impressive. But I believe it's the whole food that's important. There is still so much we don't know about how nutrients work together, versus in isolation, and so my approach is to eat what our ancestors ate: whole, real, nutrient-dense foods prepared in such a way that as much nutritional value is retained as possible.

My goal with this book is to give you what you need to know—enough to be informed, but not so much that you're overwhelmed—so that you can make better, more conscious decisions about what to eat. It's also my goal to help you start applying this information in your day-to-day life right now. Every day I work with clients who are slowly incorporating these changes into their lives. Learning what to do is one piece of the puzzle. Setting your life up to actually implement what you've learned, to create new habits, to establish new patterns—now *that* is the meat of real change. My hope is that this book will give you the tools to do just that.

For those of you who are hungry for more information, visit my website at www.eatnakednow.com for a regularly updated list of recommended reading and resources.

So, without further ado, let's take it all off...

PART 1:
the basics of eating naked

1
eat naked?

Welcome to the wonderful world of eating naked!

First, let's get one thing straight. When I say, "eat naked," I'm not talking about your clothes. I'm talking about your food. I'm talking about eating without the extras that contribute to poor health, excess weight, low energy levels, and a host of other challenges that face so many of us.

Eating naked is delicious, fun, simple, and, best of all, will make you look and feel great naked. It means eating:

- **Food that's whole, unrefined, and often comes unpackaged.** An example is eating an apple rather than a processed apple snack.

- **Food that's grown naturally.** This means it's organic and has been grown or raised (in the case of animal products) without pesticides, herbicides, antibiotics, or other synthetic chemicals at any point during growing, storage, or transport. In the case of our apple, it would be one that was grown organically.

- **Food that's fresh, in season, and ideally hasn't been preserved.** A fresh apple eaten in the fall, when it's in season, is a perfect example. If the food has been preserved for later consumption, this has been done without artificial preservatives and in a way that does the least amount of damage to the nutritional integrity of the food. Dried apple slices without any extra preservatives are a great choice.

- **Food that's grown locally.** Locally grown foods come to you without all the extra transportation miles and the associated environmental and nutritional costs. The shorter the distance the food has traveled to you, the better. An apple grown within a few hundred miles of you will be fresher, tastier, and more nutritious than an apple grown on the other side of the world, shipped great distances, and stored for months.

- **Food that's prepared minimally.** We're shooting for food enjoyed without lots of extra sauces, additives, or unhealthy fats. So often food is overprepared. Naked food isn't overcooked, which means its nutrients haven't been cooked out of it. Naked food doesn't have lots of additives and extra, unnecessary ingredients (many of which are damaging to our health) for enhanced, artificial flavoring. Naked food is prepared simply, quickly, and without all of those extras. It is delicious in its own right.

Eating naked is eating in a way that takes us back to the basics. It isn't complicated, but for many people it's a different way of eating than they've grown accustomed to. Eating naked is a paradigm shift from the commercially prepared to the homemade, a shift that yields positive results for your body, mind, and soul.

An Epiphany

Let me share an experience I had that highlighted to me the importance of eating naked. A few years back, I was invited to some friends' home for dinner. To me they represent a fairly typical middle-class American family. He runs the family business passed down from his dad; she runs the household and has a part-time marketing gig to supplement his income. They have two very active kids, both in grade school.

At their place, life feels hectic. It's obvious within moments of walking through the door that they're squeezing every last drop out of every minute of the day: school, soccer practice, piano lessons, spin class, a trip to the coast for the weekend, homework. The word "downtime" isn't part of their lingo.

As we chatted around the island in their kitchen, she was pulling together dinner. Two dinners, actually—one for the adults and one for the kids.

On the adults' menu that night was frozen broccoli and cauliflower in a cheesy cream sauce on pasta with barbecued chicken. It was a square meal of sorts—vegetables, starches, dairy, and meat—but everything came out of a bag, box, or can. To drink, they had diet cola or low-calorie beer to offer.

On the kids' menu was boxed mac and cheese with a hot dog cut into it and a couple of baby carrots on the side (left untouched). The eldest of the two sipped on a can of soda and pouted about having to eat anything at all. She pushed food around her plate so that it would look like she'd eaten some of it—enough to get excused from the table, at least. The youngest ate his meal eagerly (with the exception of the carrots), and guzzled down a big glass of strawberry-flavored drink.

When we sat down to eat, it was only a matter of minutes before the conversation turned to the litany of health challenges the family was experiencing: digestive distress, allergies, asthma, trouble sleeping, and ADHD. I watched the little girl sipping on her soda. The big, dark circles under her watchful eyes and pale, almost translucent skin seemed wrong on a girl of her age, who you'd expect to be rosy cheeked and energetic.

I left their house that night deeply disturbed. At first glance this family looks like the picture of health. None of them has weight issues, they're quite active, and they certainly fit a lot into their days. But under the surface, there were some real problems creeping up. Given my own perspective on the connections between food and health, I couldn't help but wonder whether their diet—all of which (except the carrots) was heavily processed and premade—was the root of the problem. But looking at their busy, action-packed lifestyle, it wasn't hard to see why my friends were relying on convenience foods. It was clear they were doing their best with what they knew and had available to them. And yet I wondered if there could be another way.

This isn't an unusual scenario. Families all across the United States are struggling with how to feed their families with limited time and money. I don't think it's a coincidence that so many are also struggling with serious health problems. The health statistics tell us a depressing story:

- Over 70 percent of deaths in the United States are due to a disease that can be directly related to lifestyle and, in particular, diet. This number accounts for more than two out of every three deaths, ahead of deaths by accidental causes, homicides, and an array of nonpreventable diseases (Xu et al. 2010).

- 67 percent of American adults over the age of twenty are overweight; over half of these are obese (Ogden and Carroll 2010).

- Perhaps most disturbingly, obesity rates among children are now so high that a recent study published in the *New England Journal of Medicine* shows that today's children are the first generation predicted to have a shorter life span than their parents (Olshansky et al. 2005).

It's not hard to see that these numbers affect every one of us.

These statistics are entirely unacceptable for a country that is among the wealthiest, at the cutting edge of medical research and health innovations, and with some of the most expensive and expansive health care systems on the planet.

Something doesn't fit.

Is it inevitable? Are these deaths and is this rate of sickness and disease simply part of the dues we must pay in order to maintain the standard of life to which we have become accustomed? Or is this an indicator that perhaps something has gone awry and our priorities need to be reexamined? Is it even possible to have it all? To live full, abundant lives *and* still have time for proper self-care and healthy diet choices?

I believe we can have it all. And I believe that the solution is so simple and right under our noses that we've overlooked it. I believe we need to go back to the basics. We need to take off the extras and get back to the fundamentals, especially with our food. I believe we need to eat naked.

Why Eating Naked Works

Our bodies are very, very wise. They know what they need, and they will do what they need to do to get it. Cravings, excessive appetite, and overeating are all ways our bodies communicate with us, asking for something that they're not getting but need.

When we eat foods that aren't naked—foods that have been overprocessed, that have lots of additives and little nutritional value—we aren't giving our bodies the nutritional building blocks they need to thrive. As a result, we need more food to fill that void. Typically, non-naked foods fill us, but they don't feed and nourish us.

Consider this: If you eat an apple, do you want to eat another, and another, and another? Do you have an unstoppable urge to keep eating that same food to the point of completely overstuffing yourself? No, most likely you don't. Your body takes what it needs from the apple, and then you're satisfied and don't need another apple.

Now, in comparison, consider this: If you open a bag of potato chips, do you want to eat another, and another, and another? Do you have an unstoppable urge to keep eating that same food to the point of overstuffing yourself? For many people, the answer is a resounding yes! Just as the ads proudly state, it's impossible to eat just one.

In a nutshell, eating naked means:

Shifting from...	To...
Foods that are heavily processed and refined, that contain little nutritional value and a host of unhealthy fats, sweeteners, flavorings, and chemicals to enhance flavor and extend shelf life.	Foods that are fresh and unprocessed, or in other words, whole. Or, if they've been processed, the processing has been minimal and done in such a way as to preserve the nutritional value of the food.
Food that has been prepared using low-quality ingredients and preparation methods that reduce the nutritional value of the food.	Food that is prepared minimally, using high-quality ingredients and preparation methods that preserve and sometimes even enhance the food's nutritional value.
Foods that are grown using high volumes of pesticides, herbicides, and other chemicals to ensure high yield and quick crop turnover.	Foods that are grown naturally, organically, and without pesticides, herbicides, and other chemicals.

Is this unstoppable urge the evidence of a potato chip deficiency? No, quite the opposite. Potato chips are nutritionally void and aren't giving your body what it needs. So, your body has to ask for more and more in an effort to get what it needs to be truly satisfied. In fact, the overly refined vegetable oils in potato chips block your body's ability to digest and absorb essential fatty acids, leaving your body deficient and craving more fat. As I said earlier, your body is wise—it needs fat, so it asks for fat. How we respond to what it's asking for is what makes all the difference.

The beautiful thing about eating naked is that you're giving your body what it needs to thrive. This means that you can listen to and trust your body's messages, especially when you respond to those messages with naked foods.

If your body's telling you that you're still hungry, then you're still missing something. Ignoring that message and depriving yourself is only going to trigger a stress response. Ironically, this response increases cortisol and insulin production, telling your body to store more fat—the opposite result of what most people are looking for (David 2005). Listening to your body and feeding it with nutrient-dense, whole foods truly nourishes your body, satisfies you, and helps you avoid the downward spiral of deprivation that causes most diets to fail.

Your body knows what it needs to be healthy. When you eat mostly naked foods, your body will find its natural equilibrium and you won't be tempted to overeat. Your cravings will diminish and you won't feel deprived or starved—you will be deeply nourished. When you're truly nourished, your body can find its natural, optimal health and the pounds you want to lose will go away of their own accord, without dieting.

Some Definitions

In the following chapters I'll explain specifically what eating naked means in each major food group. But first I'll define a few key terms that I'll be using.

Whole. A *whole food* means that the food is as close to its original form as possible. A great example of this is rice. Whole-grain rice or brown rice is rice that has all its parts. These include the bran, the most nutrient-rich part of the grain that contains fiber, vitamins, and minerals; the germ, which contains antioxidants and vitamins; and the endosperm, which provides energy through carbohydrates and proteins. White rice is rice that has the bran and germ removed, thus removing key components of the grain and much of its nutritional value.

Unrefined or unprocessed. Much like whole food, an *unrefined* food has had little to nothing done to change it from its original form. Continuing with the rice example, brown rice is an unrefined form of rice. Rice pasta or rice cakes have been processed into a new form.

Processed food. This is an umbrella term to describe all the different ways that food manufacturers modify raw ingredients to make food products. For example, taking tomatoes and making them into canned tomato sauce or making potatoes into potato chips or instant mashed potatoes are methods of processing the original ingredients. When I say "processed" foods, I am talking about industrial processing in which foods have been modified in such a way that we are no longer eating the whole food and its nutritional value has been compromised. This type of food processing is a development of the industrial age, which has broader priorities than simply our health. In this age, storage, transportation, market saturation, and commercial viability all trump nutritional integrity. In some cases, food processing actually creates foods that don't exist in nature and are very harmful to our bodies. High-fructose corn syrup, artificial nonsugar sweeteners, and hydrogenated oils are some of the more well-known examples of this. We'll talk more about these ingredients in the next chapter.

Preserved food. There's an important distinction between preserving food and processing food. Preservation techniques have been used for centuries to keep seasonal food available for safe consumption at other times of the year. Traditional canning, fermentation, and drying processes are examples of food preservation that maintains a great deal of the food's nutritional value. Some of these techniques (fermentation in particular) even enhance the nutritional value of the food.

Organic. This is a term used to describe food that has been grown naturally, using traditional methods, without synthetic pesticides, herbicides, genetic modification, or chemical agents.

Local. I'm considering local food to be food that has been grown within a 500-mile radius of where you're living.

In Summary

While the statistics may be grim and the outlook for the health of Americans a little dismal if we continue on our current trajectory, I believe there's a different path that's right in front of us. It's a path that's delicious, deeply nourishing, and ultimately not that difficult. This book is one step down that alternate path toward reclaiming our right to live rich, healthy, thriving lives.

2

if you're not eating naked, what are you eating?

Okay, let's get honest. When was the last time you looked in the mirror and truly felt good about what you saw? This morning? Last year? Ten years ago? Or was it when you were a little kid in your bathing suit, coming in from running through the sprinkler in your backyard on a summer afternoon, long before you were aware of such a thing as body image?

For lots of reasons, many of us struggle with loving our bodies as they are. Many of these reasons are fed by the media; some of them the result of the endless and impossible pursuit of perfection. And some of them are actually because we're eating foods that aren't working for us. Many of us are living in bodies that are rebelling by hanging on to unwanted pounds and showing all sorts of signs of unrest. Your body may not be at ease. It may, in fact, be in a state of "dis-ease." It is my belief that processed foods—foods that are most definitely not naked—are at the root of much bodily distress.

The vast majority of household food budgets in this country are spent on processed food. In fact, most of the food that lines our supermarket shelves is processed. It's not a pretty picture.

Harmful Effects of Processed Foods

So what's the big deal? How are processed foods harmful? My mother makes tomato sauce from tomatoes, you might be thinking, and instant mashed potatoes are incredibly handy. What's the problem?

Unfortunately, many processed foods, even those as harmless-seeming as canned tomato sauce, have ingredients your mom wouldn't ever use. And some of these additives have been shown to do some significant damage to our health. Here's a sampling of some of the more harmful ingredients you'll commonly find in processed foods:

- Partially or fully hydrogenated oils

- High-fructose corn syrup

- Artificial nonsugar sweeteners

- Excess sodium

- Soy, in all its many forms

- Gluten

Let's look at each of these in a little more detail.

Partially or Fully Hydrogenated Oils

Partially or fully hydrogenated oils are the dreaded "trans fats" we hear so much about. According to researchers (Mensink and Katan 1990), these fats have been shown to increase LDL and VLDL (the "bad" cholesterols) and lower HDL (the "good" cholesterol). They also contribute to a host of health problems, including obesity (Kavanagh et al. 2007), heart disease (Willett et al. 1993), diabetes (Sundram, Karupaiah, and Hayes 2007), cancer (Chajès et al. 2008), immune-system problems (Enig 2000), and reproductive challenges (Chavarro et al. 2007).

What Are Partially or Fully Hydrogenated Fats?

Hydrogenated fats are made from vegetable oils that are very unstable in their natural form, meaning they become rancid really easily. This poses transportation, storage, and shelf-life problems. To avoid these problems, food manufacturers forcibly alter the fat at the molecular level, adding hydrogen atoms to stabilize the oil. In other words, they *hydrogenate* the oil, solidifying an oil that was previously liquid at room temperature. Margarine is the classic example of a hydrogenated fat. These oils don't exist in nature, and they are unrecognizable and quite damaging to the body (Enig 2000).

Are Products Labeled "Trans-Fat Free" Okay?

Sometimes the label "trans-fat free" truly means there are no partially or fully hydrogenated oils in the product. Unfortunately, there's a loophole in the labeling laws, so you can't always be sure. The FDA labeling law allows food manufacturers to claim their products are trans-fat free as long as an individual serving of the food has less than 0.5 grams of trans fat. There are no requirements for how large the serving size is, and, of course, as soon as you eat more than one serving you may be unknowingly consuming trans fats in significant quantities. Interestingly, the Institute of Medicine (2002) has claimed that any amount of trans fat is unsafe.

The only way to be sure that you're not getting any trans fat is to scour the ingredient list on the label for partially or fully hydrogenated oils. Or skip this hassle altogether and eat naked.

High-Fructose Corn Syrup

High-fructose corn syrup has been the darling of the food-processing industry. Cheap to make and an efficient use of one of America's largest crops, high-fructose corn syrup has found its way into many of our staple food products. It's nearly ubiquitous: You'll find it in soft drinks, fruit juices, cereals, cookies, breads, sauces, dressings, flavored yogurts, peanut butter, cough syrup, processed meats, and so on. It's even in some "healthy" products like protein and energy bars.

Until the 1970s, most of the sugar we consumed came from sugarcane or sugar beets. Only in the last forty years have we have turned to corn for its sugar. This sweetener is made from cornstarch and is chemically manipulated to have high levels of fructose, accounting for its incredible sweetness (Sanda 2004). Indeed, a recent study suggested that over 10 percent of our total calories come from our consumption of fructose alone, most of which comes from sweetened beverages (Vos et al. 2008).

Why Is High-Fructose Corn Syrup So Bad?

You may be wondering why something that comes from fruit (fructose is fruit sugar, right?) can be so bad. Well, fructose *is* a naturally occurring sugar found in fruits. Most of this sugar naturally contains an approximate one-to-one ratio of fructose to glucose (in high-fructose corn syrup the ratio can be as high as four to one fructose to glucose). In a whole fruit, however, you are eating all the other micronutrients in the fruit, such as vitamins, minerals, and enzymes, along with the sugars. Also, the fiber in the fruit slows your body's metabolism of that sugar.

In the case of high-fructose corn syrup, you're missing out on the benefits of eating actual fruit. There is no fiber to slow down how quickly your body metabolizes the sugar. You aren't getting any of the other nutrients found in fruit. And, to make matters worse, consumption of high-fructose corn syrup actually depletes your body's stores of these important micronutrients, as they are required for its assimilation (Sanda 2004).

One of the many reasons high-fructose corn syrup is so hard on your health is that it's converted to fat faster than any other sugar (Parks et al. 2008). Ironically, fructose is often used as the sweetener in low-fat diet foods, achieving the very opposite of the intended result.

In addition, consuming high levels of fructose disrupts glucose metabolism. This disruption eventually leads to insulin resistance and the development of metabolic syndrome—one small step away from diabetes and cardiovascular disease (Basciano, Federico, and Adeli 2005).

Artificial, Nonsugar Sweeteners

Knowing the damage that sugar and, in particular, high-fructose corn syrup does to our system, it can be tempting to think that we're home free if we eat only sugar-free options. Unfortunately, artificial nonsugar sweeteners such as aspartame (in NutraSweet and Equal), sucralose (in Splenda), and saccharin can be even more damaging to our health than their sugar counterparts. In fact, a 2005 study done at the University of Texas Health

Science Center in San Antonio showed that drinking diet sodas increases the risk of obesity by 41 percent for every can of soda consumed daily (Fowler et al. 2008).

How Do People Get Fat from Sugar-Free Soda?

There are different theories about how sugar-free sodas lead to weight gain. One theory is that because they have no calories, those who use artificial sweeteners are more likely to assume a "free pass" and eat more overall. Another theory is that simply the taste of something sweet can lead to increased body weight due to the psychological processes initiated by that taste, even in the absence of sugar (Swithers and Davidson 2008).

Fundamentally, artificial sweeteners are man-made chemical compounds that don't exist in nature. Therefore, they are unrecognizable to our bodies, much like trans fats, and are one more burden on an often already overburdened system. Saccharin has been linked to cancer (Taylor, Weinberger, and Friedman 1980; Squire 1985) and aspartame has been linked to migraines in particular (Koehler and Glaros 1988), although complaints of a variety of health challenges due to aspartame have been reported to the FDA, from strokes, seizures, and memory loss to irritability, heart palpitations, and vertigo. In fact, over ninety different documented reactions have been reported to the FDA regarding aspartame, and yet it continues to be an approved food additive (Mercola and Pearsall 2000).

Excess Sodium

One of the easiest ways to bring out the flavor in a dish is to add salt. You might have experienced this yourself: if something tastes bland, add salt and suddenly it's tasty. Even sugar tastes sweeter if you add salt.

Well, this phenomenon isn't limited to your kitchen. Restaurants and food manufacturers have known this for a long time and make ample use of it. As a result, sodium levels in packaged, refined, processed, and restaurant foods (even those restaurants that use whole, healthy foods) are high.

Excess sodium increases blood pressure, one of the primary risk factors in heart disease, the leading cause of death in the United States. While sodium is an important mineral to include in your diet, many of us are consuming levels far higher than the FDA-recommended 2,300 milligram (mg) daily maximum. (In fact, some experts believe that even 2,300 mg is too high, recommending limits closer to 1,500 mg per day.) This overdose is often due to the high amounts of sodium in packaged and processed foods (Angell 2010). According to the American Heart Association (2010), up to 75 percent of our sodium intake comes from the consumption of processed and prepared foods.

A quick look at some common American lunches shows how far off track processed and prepared foods take us:

- According to the "Nutrition Facts" document for Denny's, the Spicy Buffalo Chicken Melt sandwich has a whopping 3,820 mg of sodium.

- Applebee's nutrition information shows the Santa Fe Chicken Salad (a salad!) has 3,420 mg of sodium.

- A cup of Campbell's Chunky Microwavable Beef with Country Vegetables soup has 890 mg of sodium, according to Campbell's nutrition facts.

These are just some examples. High sodium levels in processed and prepared foods are the norm.

One way to watch your sodium levels is to become a diligent label reader and count your sodium intake to ensure you're not exceeding the maximum. An even easier way to do this is to avoid the hassle of reading labels altogether and eat naked.

Soy, in All Its Many Forms

In recent decades, soy has become synonymous with "health food." Unfortunately, this is largely a myth perpetuated by the food industry. Traditionally grown and prepared soy is indeed a healthy food. But most of the soy in our diets is not grown or prepared using traditional methods.

Traditionally Prepared Soy

Soy wasn't originally considered a food at all. It was used in Asia as a nitrogen fixer to enhance the soil between crop rotations. It wasn't until food-preparation techniques such as fermentation were applied that it was incorporated into the human diet, and even then just in small quantities.

Soy is one of the most difficult legumes to digest, as it has powerful enzyme inhibitors. *Enzymes* are some of the natural chemicals the body uses to break down the foods we eat. As the name implies, an enzyme inhibitor makes it harder for our body to break down food. Fermentation processes neutralize these enzyme inhibitors, making traditional soy foods such as miso, tempeh, and natto much easier to digest. (See chapter 14, "Better Than Naked," for more information on fermentation.) While these forms of soy do exist in the American diet, they account for a tiny portion of the soy we consume.

Soy in the American Diet

In our diet, soy appears most often broken down into isolated components: soybean oil, soy protein isolates, soy isoflavones, and soy lecithin are just some examples. You may think you don't eat a diet heavy in soy, especially if you're not a vegetarian. But once you start looking under the surface, soy is hiding in many processed foods and in places you'd find highly unlikely. You'll find soy in meats (yes, meats—as a filler), salad dressings, low-carb versions of high-carb foods, cereals, and many other processed foods.

The reason for this is that soy is an extremely cheap and abundant source of protein. Second only to corn, soy is one of the largest crops produced by the United States. In the 1950s, the food industry had a waste problem on their hands: Soy oil was used extensively in processed foods, which left the remaining components of the soybean, namely the protein, as waste. Waste wasn't an attractive option, so food processors began to aggressively market soy protein as a healthy, vegetarian substitute for meat and dairy to the health conscious (Daniel 2005).

Antinutrients in Soy

Were the soybean as innocuous as it sounds, using this natural protein would be a great alternative to eating animal products. Unfortunately, there are many "antinutrients" present in soy that make it less than ideal, the enzyme inhibitors mentioned above being one example. Soy also contains *oxalates* and *phytates*, two compounds that block the body's ability to absorb vital minerals, such as calcium, zinc, and iron. Soy also delivers *isoflavones*, or phytoestrogens, estrogen-mimicking plant hormones that affect the reproductive system in both men and women. Soy is also one of

21

the top eight food allergens (Mayo Clinic Staff 2009), and has *goitrogens*, which have been shown to damage the thyroid (Daniel 2005).

Gluten

Gluten, the protein in wheat, rye, and barley, is fast becoming another top allergen. Gluten intolerance can show up in a number of different ways. It may present as a food sensitivity, in which your system is overburdened by a specific food and reacts adversely to it when consumed. You may develop a full-blown allergy to gluten, in which your system mounts an immune response to the protein when you consume it. The reactions to a gluten allergy can be so intense as to constitute a disease—celiac disease, an autoimmune disorder in which the villi of the small intestine are damaged by the gluten protein. Although this condition was originally thought to be rare, the website of Celiac Disease Center at Columbia University Medical Center estimates one in 133 people in the United States has celiac disease, many cases of which remain undiagnosed.

Gluten Intolerance

Many people don't know they're sensitive to gluten, so their symptoms of intolerance or allergy are not recognized as such. For example, after eating do you ever experience headaches, fatigue, foggy thinking, irritability, or digestive distress, such as bloating, gas, cramps, or unexplained diarrhea? Did you know that these are all symptoms of gluten intolerance? Many people just live with these symptoms. In many ways, they are so prevalent in our society that we have come to normalize them. I have seen many clients, even those who aren't formally diagnosed with gluten intolerance, thrive and experience significant health improvements when they eliminate gluten from their diet.

Gluten Dominance

Gluten is problematic in processed foods because it is so prevalent. Aside from wheat, rye, and barley, and the obvious products made from them such as breads, pastas, cereals, baked goods, and beer, gluten hides in unlikely places such as salad dressings, gravies, and sauces (as a thickening agent), as well as seasonings, prepared meats, candies, chocolate bars, some nutritional supplements, medications, and beauty products. I can remember sitting at lunch one day with a good friend who has a severe gluten allergy. She grabbed my lip gloss and put some on, and then casually read the ingredients on the label—only to be horrified at seeing gluten among them. Thank goodness there were some sturdy cloth napkins on hand so she could wipe the gloss off before it did any damage.

To be truly gluten free means to diligently inquire about ingredients when eating out at restaurants and to scour labels for the long list of gluten-containing substances when eating any processed or pre-prepared foods.

Or, as you might have guessed by now, you can skip this altogether by eating naked, eliminating many of the gluten-containing products from your grocery list and making gluten-free living a much simpler prospect.

In Summary

You may be wondering at this point why on earth all this health-damaging stuff is in our processed foods. Well, each ingredient I've listed has properties that either extend shelf life, bind food, enhance flavor, alter the nutritional makeup, or otherwise add to the commercial viability of the food. The key word here, of course, is "commercial." When food is processed, its economics take center stage and overshadow priorities such as the health and nutritional integrity of what we're eating.

Label reading can truly be crazy making. I still need to do it sometimes, and it's no fun. I believe there is a simpler way, and that's to avoid processed foods and the hassles of label reading—altogether by eating naked.

3
why eat naked?

Now that we've gone through some of the uglier sides of eating non-naked foods, we can see that processed and prepared foods aren't ideal. Is eating naked so much better?

Yes! And for lots of reasons.

You'll Give Your Body What It Needs

Your body is very wise. It knows what it needs, and it's going to ask for more until it gets it. When you eat food that is nutrient rich and power-fully nourishing, your body doesn't need as much of it to feel full and to get the nutritional value that it requires. If you're eating really low-quality food that's basically nutritionally void, your body is going to keep asking for more and more food, looking for the nutrients it's missing (David 2005).

I have experienced this myself quite powerfully. I used to be what I call a "junk-food vegetarian," eating lots of highly processed foods. I was known among my friends for my insatiable appetite. I could eat and eat and eat and never feel satisfied. I would be full—in fact, sometimes my stomach would be distended from the volumes of food I'd crammed into it—but I was still hungry.

When I changed my diet to include truly whole foods that were nutri-ent dense, suddenly I wasn't insatiable anymore. I could eat about a third of what I'd eaten previously and feel not only full, but deeply satisfied. It was quite an amazing change. I've tested my theory and eaten nutritionally depleted, highly processed foods, and guess what? My insatiable appetite returned.

You'll Lose That Extra Weight

So, we've seen that if you're giving your body the nutrition it requires, it doesn't need to eat as much. You can probably guess what that means for your waistline. By eating whole foods, your appetite will regulate to an appropriate level for your body and the weight can shift of its own accord, without dieting. This is a really nice side benefit of eating naked.

Also, recall the negative impacts of some of the common ingredients in non-naked foods we talked about in the last chapter. Artificial non-sugar sweeteners trigger the fat-storage mechanism in your body even in the absence of an increase in blood sugar levels. Fructose gets converted to fat at a faster rate than do other sugars, making high-fructose corn syrup a fat-creating ingredient even in "low-fat" foods. Hydrogenated oils, unrec-ognizable to the body, actually block your body's ability to use and absorb the essential fatty acids you need, increasing cravings for fat.

The simplest way to avoid these fat-increasing responses in your body is to eat naked and avoid introducing these ingredients into your body's chemistry to begin with.

You Are What You Eat

Let's say weight isn't an issue for you. Is eating naked still important?

It's a cliché, but it's true: we are what we eat. Take a moment and look at your hand. Think of the miraculous machine that it is; notice the finely articulated bones, muscles, tendons, fingernails, blood, and skin. All of that was once food. Every little bit of it. As Joshua Rosenthal so aptly said, "We are, at our most basic level, walking food" (Rosenthal 2008, 234). So, do you want those building blocks to come from a basket of cheesy chili fries or something a little higher quality? If you bought a brand new Porsche, would you put supersaver gas in it?

When you're eating nutrient-dense foods, you're giving your body the building blocks it needs. This means it has a much better ability to heal if you're unwell, to stay healthy when you get there, and to truly thrive.

One of the pioneers in the field of nutrition, Dr. Weston A. Price, discovered how very powerful it is to eat a nutrient-dense diet. Dr. Price set about investigating the diets of indigenous peoples, trying to determine whether these traditional ways of choosing, preparing, and eating food impacted the health of those he encountered. He was curious to discover whether people in these cultures experienced better health, and if so, if there were common factors in their diets.

He found that "beautiful straight teeth, freedom from decay, good physiques, resistance to disease, and fine characters were typical of native groups on their traditional diets, rich in essential nutrients" (Weston A. Price Foundation 2000, 2). Not surprisingly, these diets were completely free of any kind of industrially processed foods. The Weston A. Price Foundation summarizes the diets he found in their *Principles of Healthy Diets* booklet:

> The diets of healthy, nonindustrialized peoples contain no refined or denatured foods or ingredients, such as refined sugar or high-fructose corn syrup; white flour; canned foods; pasteurized, homogenized, skim, or low-fat milk; refined or hydrogenated vegetable oils; protein powders; synthetic vitamins, or toxic additives and artificial colorings. (2000, 4)

Discussing epidemiological studies on populations that consumed nutrient-rich, "naked" foods, nutritionist George Mateljan notes that such a diet may result in "a considerably lower risk of developing many chronic degenerative diseases, including cardiovascular disease, type 2 diabetes, cancer, rheumatoid arthritis, Alzheimer's disease and depression" (Mateljan 2007, 72).

It's Delicious

Aside from the health benefits, there are lots of other reasons to eat naked. For one, contrary to popular misconception, eating healthy doesn't have to be tasteless. In fact, it's one of the most delicious ways to eat. Food that's processed often has the flavor cooked out of it—part of the reason for the artificial flavoring, added sodium, and other creative ways food manufacturers have found to make food that can live on your shelf for years and still taste like food.

Eating fresh food is simply delicious. You might have had the luxury of eating an egg from a local farm where the chickens are left to wander freely and are fed diets they're biologically designed to eat. Maybe it was even an egg that was laid that morning, cooked in a little organic butter from grass-fed cows. Scrumptious! What a different taste and experience from eating an egg that comes from a factory farm and is shipped across the country, weeks old, and cooked in a microwave into an un-egg shape, then put inside a soggy, refined-flour English muffin.

Typically, the more naked a food, the yummier it is. Enough said. Check out the recipes in chapter 13 to judge for yourself.

It's Simple

Eating healthy doesn't have to be hard or complicated. All it takes is a few basic principles and a new way of looking at the food you eat.

As you saw in the previous chapter, eating healthy becomes much more difficult when you try to do so with processed foods. In order to eat healthfully *and* eat processed food, you must become an expert label reader. You need to be versed in the most recent nutrition labeling laws, which ingredients may be harmful, and the various names and forms under which unhealthful ingredients are listed. I have heard some of the most seasoned nutritionists exclaim their frustration at deciphering labels. It can be a maddening exercise. And really, who has the time?

Eating naked skips this step altogether. If you don't eat processed food, basically you're not eating food that comes with lots of mysterious and unpronounceable ingredients. Often you're eating food that comes unpackaged, so there's no label to read. Much, much simpler and much, much faster.

It's a Lifestyle

Eating naked isn't a fad diet. It's the way we ate for thousands of years, before the advent of processed food. It simply means eating real food and is a step toward simplicity and back to the basics.

Many diets require significant deprivation along with complicated premises, strict rules, and endless calories or points to count. It's well-known that most people who lose weight on a weight-loss diet gain the full amount back within a couple of years, and the high maintenance level of most diets is a big component of such incredibly low success rates. Aside from being difficult, unsatisfying, and unsustainable for most people, this approach takes so much of the joy out of eating.

Eating naked is something for the whole family. It's not "Mom on a diet" while the rest of the family goes about their business. It's an optimal way of eating for everyone, no matter what age, stage of life, or particular health concern.

It's Good for the World

Eating naked isn't just good for you, your waistline, your health, and your enjoyment of your dinner. Eating naked is a powerful way to be environmentally responsible and support your local economy.

Many industrial food-manufacturing techniques, from the growing to the processing and transportation of our food, are harmful to the environment. Toxic runoff from feedlot farms, the use of pesticides and herbicides, and the carbon emissions from transporting food such long distances are just some of the environmental challenges we hear about in the news on a regular basis. Furthermore, these practices can be harmful to farmworkers. Pesticides have been shown to create health problems in fieldworkers, and some of the most dangerous jobs are those in industrial slaughterhouses. By choosing naked foods, you're not only taking care of your own health, you're also supporting a healthier environment for those who've produced the food.

Shifting away from industrial-scale to more local produce also means supporting businesses in your area. Not only is the food fresher (having traveled a shorter distance to get to your plate), you're able to give local farmers and food vendors your spending dollars. It's like effecting your own economic stimulus plan right in your backyard.

Eating naked is as good for the health of the planet and the economy as it is for you.

It's a Truly Long-Term Solution

As humans, we're biologically wired to seek pleasure and avoid pain. Eating is one way we can satisfy that need for pleasure, and it's something we do multiple times every day. Eating can be one of the most deeply pleasurable and sensual experiences. When was the last time you really, thoroughly enjoyed a meal without any feeling of guilt? It's not something we allow ourselves to do very often, and our relationship with food becomes one of control and willpower. The more we deprive ourselves of that pleasure, the more we want it—and the more unsustainable the deprivation approach will be.

Eating naked is about getting back into that place of joy and pleasure with our food. When you're eating naked, you can breathe easy, relax into your meal, and know that you're being really good to your body while eating delicious food. Eating naked isn't about deprivation, about counting calories, grams, or points, or about any other tedious, time-consuming, and difficult restrictions. And because eating naked isn't about deprivation, focusing instead on honoring our body's deep and primal need for pleasure, it's a truly long-term solution that doesn't rest on willpower and overcoming natural urges.

In Summary

Eating naked is good for you and your family, as well as the health of the environment, your local economy, and the people who produce your food. It's delicious, and once you get familiar with the basic principles, it's not that hard to do. Let's shift gears now and look at what eating naked means specifically for different types of food.

4
naked produce

I love vegetables. I really do. I'm not saying that to impress you or to scare you. I'm just stating the fact: I really love vegetables. I was that weird breed of kid who ate my broccoli first and mashed potatoes second, and pushed my meat around the plate trying to make it get small so my parents wouldn't notice I hadn't eaten it.

Now, let me be specific. I don't love *all* vegetables. A dry, tasteless tomato shipped thousands of miles in mid-January is not my idea of delicious. The kind of tomato I'm talking about is one eaten in the middle of summer when they're in season, grown nearby, maybe even from my little patio garden. It's a small gem, picked fresh and ripe, juicy, impossibly sweet, with flavor bursting out of it. Sliced thick, with a few sprigs of fresh basil, some olive oil, and a little balsamic vinegar drizzled on top—now *that's* a tomato.

Vegetables are the cornerstone of a naked diet. There's a reason your mother used to nag you about eating your veggies. They're really good for you! Vegetables and fruit are chock-full of vitamins, minerals, fiber, and an awe-inspiring array of potent *antioxidants* (powerful little agents that help mitigate the negative effects of food breaking down, or *oxidation*, and the production of cell-damaging free radicals).

The gold standard when it comes to naked produce is:

- Local (grown within five hundred miles or less of your home)

- In season (this will usually go hand-in-hand with local)

- Fresh (in other words, not processed and usually not frozen or canned)

- Organic (grown without chemicals or genetic modifications)

Now, it's obvious that meeting all of these criteria every time isn't possible. But when it is—in the spring, summer, and fall in most places in North America—I highly recommend you go for it.

Organic: To Be or Not to Be?

Is organically grown produce more nutritious, better for you, and ultimately healthier than industrially grown produce? There has been lots of debate over this. Unsurprisingly, producers of conventionally grown vegetables and fruit have gone to great lengths to show that there are few nutritional benefits to consuming organic rather than conventional produce. However, there has been ample evidence that the nutritional value of produce grown organically is greater than its conventionally grown counterparts (Worthington 2001; Mitchell et al. 2007). I believe the issue is much broader than the considerations of nutrition, so let me share some of the reasons why I believe it's important to eat organic.

For the soil. The quality of our soil is slowly deteriorating. In traditional farming, before the advent of chemical fertilizers and herbicides, farmers used crop rotation to ensure sustainably rich soil. Different crops pull different nutrients from the soil, and some crops replenish the soil's nutrient stores (remember from chapter 2 that soy was originally grown for its ability to fix nitrogen in the soil). Conventional, industrial farming techniques favor monocrops (the practice of growing the same crop on the same land year after year) and pursue high yields. These factors require aggressive pesticide and fertilizer use that ultimately depletes rather than replenishes the soil. On the other hand, organic farming builds up organic matter in the soil. This process improves overall soil quality, which improves the quality of the food grown, and ultimately benefits the farmers and the environment.

For our health. For all the debate about whether pesticides affect the nutritional value of a food, there is little doubt that they negatively affect our health when consumed. After all, the whole purpose of pesticides is to kill. The Environmental Protection Agency lists 175 chemical pesticides that are confirmed, likely, or probable carcinogens or have "suggestive evidence of carcinogenic potential" (2009, 8–17). Interestingly, all research on the health effects of pesticides has been done on each chemical in isolation. To date, no research has been done on what happens synergistically when more than one is used at a time. But we can assume that using multiple chemical compounds at once, as often happens, doesn't make the food healthier.

For the health of our farmers. If pesticides are harmful in the trace amounts found in the produce when it gets to our kitchen, it's nothing compared to the effects on the health of the farmers and laborers who are working with these substances on a daily basis. Pesticide use has been shown to damage the health of the farmers growing produce, and perhaps even more tragically, the health of their children (Flower et al. 2004). Perhaps you've noticed the smell when walking through the pesticide aisle at your local garden store. It's enough to make you gag or even feel faint. Imagine working with these chemicals in large volumes day in and day out. I don't want those who are producing my food to get ill as a result of their efforts.

For the environment. On conventional farms, pesticides and synthetic fertilizers wash away in the rain, polluting nearby streams and rivers and harming local wildlife (U.S. Geological Survey 1999). Organic farming doesn't have this problem with runoff, and it doesn't rely on petroleum-based fertilizers. This means it reduces our reliance on fossil fuels. Interestingly, recent research has shown that organic farming practices actually sequester carbon dioxide, making it a component of climate-change mitigation (LaSalle and Hepperly 2008).

Prioritize Local Foods

When it comes to produce, if you have to choose between local and organic, which would I recommend? Local. Surprised? Well, I recommend this for several reasons.

The nutritional value of local produce is greater than produce that's been shipped long distances because local produce is fresher. Vegetables and fruits that are shipped long distances might have been grown without pesticides, chemical fertilizers, genetic modification, or irradiation, but they are usually picked before they're ripe, which negatively impacts both nutritional content and flavor.

Eating locally means boosting your local economy by supporting smaller-scale farmers, many of whom are on the path to being organic even if they're not yet fully certified. It also means that the produce doesn't need to travel as far, which is significant since one of the biggest ways our food consumption affects environmental issues is through transportation. Ultimately, local eating shows support for a food economy that is much more sustainable in the long term than the large-scale industrial model we're currently using.

Keep It in Season, Within Reason

A longtime friend and resident of some of Canada's most remote northeast regions reminded me that buying local and in season isn't always entirely possible. Eating locally and seasonally is clearly a far easier feat for me, living in southern California, than for her. Where I live, farmers can grow all year long. In far northeastern Canada, the growing season is only a few short months of the year and the most abundant crop is potato. She has a point.

So, what to do when you live somewhere with long, cold winters and a short growing season? Well, the first thing to do is to make sure you're eating locally and in season when you can: in the spring, summer, and fall.

In the winter, when locally grown produce simply isn't an option, there are several things you can do.

Buy fall and winter produce. This includes root vegetables, squashes, apples, and pears, which last for weeks if stored properly.

Buy your produce frozen, ideally organic. Flash-freezing produce is one of the best ways to preserve its nutritional value. Some would argue that there's more nutritional value in frozen produce than fresh, since 'the produce is typically frozen very shortly after it's picked, and fresh produce can go for weeks between being picked and landing in your kitchen. When buying frozen produce, the most important thing is that there are no extras added: no sauces, flavors, sugar, preservatives, sodium…nothing but the fruit or vegetable.

EAT NAKED ON A BUDGET

If you need to prioritize your food dollars, buy conventionally grown produce rather than organic, and spend your organic food dollars on really high-quality fats and proteins. Toxins accumulate in fat, and thus it's most important to ensure your fats and proteins (which contain more fat than produce) are of the highest quality.

If you want to eat some of your produce organic but don't have the budget to eat all organic, spend the extra money on the fruits and vegetables that tend to be highest in pesticides. Here are the top most contaminated and least contaminated, according to the Environmental Working Group's *2010 Shopper's Guide to Pesticides*:

Dirty Dozen Buy These Organic	Clean Fifteen Lowest in Pesticides
Celery	Onions
Peaches	Avocados
Strawberries	Sweet corn (frozen)
Apples	Pineapples
Blueberries	Mangoes
Nectarines	Sweet peas (frozen)
Sweet bell peppers	Asparagus
Spinach	Kiwifruit
Kale or collard greens	Cabbage
Cherries	Eggplant
Potatoes	Cantaloupe
Grapes (imported)	Watermelon
	Grapefruit
	Sweet potatoes
	Honeydew melon

With the exception of tomatoes, stay away from canned produce. Commercial canning techniques deplete most of the nutrients from canned vegetables, and canned fruit typically comes in syrupy water. If you've ever canned your own fruit, you know that the secret is lots and lots of sugar. Far better to go with frozen fruit without any sugar added. The fruit has enough sugar all on its own.

Tomatoes, on the other hand, have a nutrient called *lycopene*, a powerful antioxidant that has been linked to reduced risk of cardiovascular disease (Mateljan 2007). Heat increases the bioavailability of lycopene, which means that your body can access and use it much more easily from cooked tomatoes than from raw ones. The canning process involves quite a lot of heat, which increases the amount of lycopene your body can get from the tomatoes. They're the one exception, but as always, be sure to get just the plain tomatoes without anything extra added in.

In the cold of winter, is it okay to eat an avocado from Mexico once in a while? Of course it is. Just prioritize the truly naked produce, making exceptions now and again as a treat.

Eat by the Rainbow

One of the simplest ways to mix it up with your vegetables is to eat a wide variety of colors. Every different color represents a different mix of antioxidants, each of which has a slightly different health benefit. For example, the antioxidant nasunin protects cells from oxidative damage and gives eggplant its deep, dark purple. Lycopene, the antioxidant in tomatoes I mentioned earlier, also gives several red and pink foods, such as watermelon and pink grapefruit, their coloring.

An easy rule of thumb is to have at least one green vegetable and then a couple of other colors on your plate. Get creative! See how colorful you can get. I often design a meal with color as a key factor.

When in Doubt, Eat More Vegetables

"How many vegetables should I eat?" is a question I get asked all the time by my clients. My answer: as many as possible. When in doubt, fill your plate with more vegetables. You really can't overdo it. In fact, most of us underdo it and need to catch up a bit.

An easy rule of thumb is to fill at least half your plate with vegetables (things other than potatoes—let's diversify from the potato, shall we?). A nice big salad is an easy one, or some steamed veggies that are in season. Or you can make a few different vegetable side dishes and have them in the fridge ready to fill out a meal at a moment's notice. Check out some of the salads and sides recipes in chapter 13 for some new ideas.

Also, you'll notice that I'm talking much more about vegetables than fruit. Certainly, fruits are also packed with good vitamins, minerals, antioxidants, and fiber. In my experience, though, fruit's natural sweetness makes it an easy thing to reach for. Most people I've worked with eat far more fruit in a day than vegetables. Generally, I recommend that you have one to two pieces of fresh fruit a day, and then vegetables with at least two if not three meals per day. If pressed to choose between vegetables and fruit, I would always pick vegetables. That's because they contain all the vitamins, minerals, and other micronutrients of fruit, with more protein, vitamin B, and the fat-soluble vitamins A and K. But really, you want to have both in your diet.

A Note on Juicing

We'll talk more about juicing and juices in chapter 10, "Naked Beverages, Sweeteners, and Condiments," but I want to make a quick point about it here while we're on the subject of produce. Generally speaking, I'm not a fan of commercial juices. Here's why.

Let's take your standard glass of orange juice as an example. If you were to sit down and eat an orange, you'd probably eat just one, maybe two if they were particularly fresh and you were particularly hungry.

When juice is made, manufacturers squeeze out and retain the water, sugar, and nutrients, leaving behind most of the fiber. Then they pasteurize the juice, heating it temporarily to destroy any possible pathogens. Unfortunately, delicate nutrients are also damaged in the process, significantly reducing nutritional value.

EAT NAKED ON A BUDGET: GARDEN NAKED

A great way to have some of the most truly naked produce right at your doorstep is to plant a garden. This can be as small as a little herb box on your windowsill or a small corner of your backyard dedicated to a few choice veggies, or a more ambitious project of growing many of your own vegetables and fruits. Growing your own veggies has many benefits. For one, the nutritional value of a vegetable is at its peak when it's just been picked, so you'll be getting nutrient-packed produce. Done properly, growing your own can end up being far cheaper than buying from the store, and you can get higher quality for lower cost. Also, you can grow your favorites or prioritize those things that are much more expensive in the stores but really easy to grow (like basil, for example). And clearly, growing your own produce is as local, in season, and fresh as you can get.

To make that one glass of juice, you need to squeeze anywhere from three to eight oranges, depending on the size and juiciness of the oranges. That's a whole lot of sugar to ingest without the fiber necessary to slow down its absorption into your body.

Essentially, you're getting a nutritionally depleted, high-sugar drink. If you really want to drink juice, my recommendation is to juice it yourself. Drink the homemade juice immediately so it doesn't have a chance to spoil and to get maximum nutritional benefit from it.

The Farmers' Market Challenge

Getting tired of the same old vegetables? So many of us get into ruts with our food. We're creatures of habit, and we tend to reach for the familiar. This can take the fun out of eating and prevent us from trying things that may have delicious surprises in store.

As we'll talk about in chapter 12, one of the best places to find naked foods is your local farmers' market. This is also a great place to break out of your vegetable and fruit habits, and to discover yummy local gems you might not even know are there. The next time you go to your local farmers' market (or wherever you get your produce), find something you either don't recognize or have never tried before. Ask the person at the booth how to prepare it. Often the vendors at farmers' markets are full of great information and are very interested in sharing as much as they can about their products. If you're buying from a grocer and there's no one to ask, look it up on the Internet when you get home for ideas.

Experimenting at a farmers' market is how I discovered the delicious vegetable kohlrabi. I had heard of it but didn't really know what it was or how to prepare it. Turns out it's delicious in stir-fries, lightly steamed with other seasonal veggies, or even grated raw into a salad.

Get adventurous. You never know what new family favorite you might discover.

In Summary

Naked produce is delicious, nutritious, and can be a great source of creative inspiration for your meals. Experiment! Check out the recipes in chapter 13, "Cook Naked," to get started, and make it your initial goal to fill up half your plate with veggies at each meal.

Produce: Good, Better, Best	
Best	Local, in season, fresh, organic
Next best	Local, in season, fresh
Okay	Frozen and organic without the extras: no sauces, flavorings, additives, or preservatives
Steer clear	Frozen with the extras, canned (except tomatoes), otherwise packaged and processed

5
naked meat

When people first learn that I'm "into nutrition," many immediately assume that means I'm a vegetarian. When they learn that I eat meat, even red meat (gasp!), their reaction usually falls somewhere between surprise and shock. (Just wait until they find out I eat butter.)

Choosing whether to eat meat is complex and ultimately very personal. My goal in this chapter is *not* to tell you that you should or should not eat meat. Some people thrive on a vegetarian diet; others need to consume meat to feel healthy. We are all unique, and our bodies need different things. Only you can make the decision, listening to your body and what it's asking for.

My goal is to help you make good choices with your meat consumption, should you choose to eat meat. These are choices that will support your health, animal welfare, and the environment. I believe there is a way to consume meat that supports all of these things.

My History with Meat

As I've shared already, I was a vegetarian (albeit not a very good one) for years. Originally I chose this way of eating for health reasons. New dietary fads were vegetarian, and I liked how pure and radical they sounded. This was during my university years, and I was newly exposed to the issues around animal welfare and environmental degradation that were associated with meat production. Learning about these issues added to my conviction and turned a health decision into a political statement. Very occasionally, I would indulge in a little meat—the occasional piece of chicken or a hamburger—but I always felt guilty about it.

I can remember reading John Robbins's *Diet for a New America* (1987) and crying myself to sleep at the horrors of animal cruelty on factory farms and the sickening tales from the slaughterhouse floor. Just looking at meat was disgusting to me, and I couldn't eat any without feeling rotten about myself and the system I was supporting through my food choices. The great problem was that my body felt amazing when I ate meat. Without it, I was insatiable and renowned for my voracious appetite; with a little meat, I needed very little food to fill me, and I had lots of energy that seemed to last and last. What a quandary.

At the time, I chose a strategy of mind over body. The arguments against meat consumption were so compelling that I disregarded my body's requests and only indulged, guiltily, on occasion. It wasn't until years later when I studied nutrition and learned about traditional farming practices that I gave my body permission to have the meat it seemed to really like and want. When I learned that there could be a way to eat meat and feel good about it, I was skeptical but open to learning more. I discovered a whole world (if still a relatively small one) of farmers who are actually contributing to environmental regeneration, who are raising animals ethically and humanely, and who are providing sources of meat that have nutritional profiles vastly superior to what we find in meat from conventionally raised animals.

What's the Problem, Anyway?

Let's first look at the issues associated with meat consumption. There are some valid and important concerns pertaining to raising animals for our food supply that deserve our attention and thoughtful consideration.

Health Issues

From a health perspective, the arguments against meat consumption are compelling. The primary argument is that meat, in particular red meat, is high in saturated fat and cholesterol. Eating too much of either has been linked to obesity, heart disease, and a host of other serious health ailments. Because meat is relatively high in fat, it tends to concentrate the pesticides, toxins, antibiotics, and growth hormones used when raising animals en masse, as many of these substances tend to accumulate in fat. Furthermore, the poor health standards maintained by many feedlots and slaughterhouses create a breeding ground for harmful bacteria to infect the meat, thus increasing the likelihood of illness from consuming contaminated meat. *E. coli* and *Salmonella* are just two of the more common examples of this type of contamination.

Addressing These Concerns

When it comes to eating meat from conventionally raised animals (those that spent much of their lives in overcrowded confinement operations or feedlots), I think many of these concerns are valid. Animals raised this way are:

- Taken out of their natural environment

- Fed food they wouldn't consume if left to their own devices

- Pumped up on growth hormones to artificially speed their development

- Given high doses of antibiotics to manage the health ailments resulting from living in such close quarters with hundreds, if not thousands, of other animals

Given these circumstances, the quality of the meat itself is invariably compromised and not a healthful food choice.

I would never encourage you to consume this kind of meat. In fact, I'd encourage you to stay far, far away from it. From the perspective of your health (we'll talk about the animal's health in a moment), the nutritional profile of industrially raised animals is significantly different from that of animals raised in their natural environments. Beef from cows raised on pasture is far lower in fat overall and has the proper ratio of omega-3 to omega-6 fatty acids (approximately one to one). Also, pasture-raised

43

beef is a source of *conjugated linoleic acid* (CLA). This important omega-6 fatty acid helps promote a healthy weight, can help lower your level of *triglycerides,* or stored fat (Blankson et al. 2000), and has been linked to cancer prevention (Belury 2002). This potentially powerful fatty acid is barely evident in feedlot beef (Dhiman et al. 1999). Cattle raised largely on pasture are much leaner and healthier, and, as a result, so is the meat that comes from them. Indeed, it was for the very purpose of fattening up the cows that we originally brought them indoors and started feeding them grains. Grass-fed beef also has more vitamin E and beta-carotene (Smith et al. 1996).

We'll explore the topic of saturated fats and cholesterol more in chapter 8, but for now I do want to be clear that I do not join those who demonize saturated fats and cholesterol as the source of so many health challenges. Both, when consumed in moderation, are vital components to a healthy diet. But, in the context of meat, they are only healthy when from an animal raised in a traditional environment. Toxins and pesticides do tend to accumulate in fatty tissue, and so the quality of the meat is vitally important. We don't want there to be pesticides, growth hormones, antibiotics, and other contaminants present to begin with, and when animals are raised using traditional farming practices, they aren't.

The Treatment of Animals

The topic of animal cruelty and the often horrifying treatment of animals destined for human consumption is one that can turn the stomach of even the most dedicated meat lover. Maybe you've seen the videos, heard the gut-wrenching stories, or read about the atrocious environments in which animals are raised and slaughtered. From chicken debeaking to cows standing knee-deep in their own manure to pigs so traumatized they tear off each other's tails, the picture isn't pretty. It's deeply disturbing, and rightfully so. Who would wish such inhumane treatment on a creature who will ultimately be sacrificing its life to feed and nurture us? If you've ever seen footage from inside a factory farm, you know the horrors that I'm talking about. The list of abominations is long and sickening.

Addressing These Concerns

Consuming meat does not necessarily require that you support this inhumane treatment of animals. One of the really nice things about eating meat from animals raised traditionally is that, in the majority of cases, the animals are coming from a smaller farm, typically a farm where they are treated well and living, by all accounts, good and happy lives. Now, can animal cruelty happen on a small family farm that raises animals traditionally? Absolutely. But it's far less likely than in massive industrial facilities where volume, efficiency, and the bottom line take precedence over the health and welfare of the animals themselves.

The only truly foolproof way to ensure that the meat on your dinner plate came from an animal that was treated humanely is to visit the farm on which it was raised. Since this isn't realistic for many of us with busy urban lives, the next best thing is to look for humane treatment certification labels. The best example of this is the Certified Humane label by the Humane Farm Animal Care organization, which certifies that rigorous standards were used in caring for the animals. These standards include allowing the animals to express natural behaviors, like chickens dust bathing, pigs rooting, and cows grazing. A next-best certification to look for is the U. S. Department of Agriculture (USDA) Certified Organic label. While organic standards don't specify humane treatment of the animal, new guidelines implemented in 2010 require that farm animals have access to pasture, which addresses at least part of the concern (U. S. Department of Agriculture 2006).

If you're buying your meat from the farmers' market and it's not certified organic or certified humane, that doesn't mean the animals were treated poorly. You can always use the old-fashioned, very low-tech way of learning more about where your food is coming from—ask. Farmers at farmers' markets are often delighted to talk about their practices, and you can always ask if you can come for a visit (even if you never intend to do so). Their willingness to show you their facilities is a good indicator of the integrity of their practices.

The Environmental Sustainability of
Meat Production

Raising animals for meat, dairy, and eggs is a major environmental challenge. As authors of the United Nations report *Livestock's Long Shadow* explain, this sector is "one of the top two or three most significant contributors to the most serious environmental problems, at every scale from local to global" (Steinfeld et al. 2006, xx). This is disconcerting, to say the least.

Industrial production of meat leads to the deforestation and clearing of wildlands to make room for the animals and, more significantly, the pasture required to grow feed crops. This speaks to the inefficiency of eating an animal versus eating the grains used to feed the animal. I've read estimates that it takes from seven to twenty pounds of grain to produce a single pound of beef (Keith 2009). That's not a lot of return on the investment of grain. In a world where hunger is still an enormous concern and the amount of arable land is decreasing annually due to soil erosion and overgrazing, the inefficiency seems preposterous. Why eat the protein and fat from an animal when we could eat what the animal ate to create our own protein and fat?

Another significant impact of industrial meat production is its contribution to climate change. You may be surprised, as I was, to learn that the livestock sector alone is responsible for 18 percent of the world's greenhouse gas emissions. This is a greater amount than even the transportation sector, the usual suspect when it comes to climate change (Steinfeld et al. 2006). The high emissions are due to a combination of the changes in land use I mentioned above, the off-gassing of manure "lagoons" (which are the industrial solution to having simply too much manure), and what's called *enteric fermentation*, a fancy term for cow burps (and buffalo, sheep, and goat burps) that release methane during the digestion process.

Further, the livestock sector is one of the largest causes of water pollution. Water sources are contaminated by animal wastes, antibiotics, growth hormones, and the pesticide residues from the crops used to feed the animals. In the United States alone, "livestock are responsible for an estimated 55 percent of erosion and sediment, 37 percent of pesticide use, 50 percent of antibiotic use, and a third of the loads of nitrogen and phosphorus into freshwater resources" (Steinfeld et al. 2006, xxii).

Addressing These Concerns

While the livestock sector is a major contributor to environmental challenges, it also has the potential to be a major contributor to environmental solutions. Once again, the question is about scale and farming methods, not simply the act of raising animals in and of itself. In fact, traditional farming practices, where the animals are integrated into the fabric of the farm, are truly sustainable and actually beneficial to the environment. As author Anna Lappé shares, "Historically, properly grazed livestock produced numerous benefits to the land: hooves aerate soil, allowing more oxygen in the ground, which helps plant growth; their hoof action also presses grass seed into the earth, fostering plant growth, too; and, of course, their manure provides natural fertilizer" (Lappé 2009, 111).

With the exception of the greenhouse gases resulting from enteric fermentation (a natural and unavoidable part of all ruminants' digestion process), all of the environmental devastations I mentioned above pertain to feedlot situations, not traditional farming practices, and largely come back to feeding the animals grain rather than what they're biologically designed to eat. The assertion that it takes seven to twenty pounds of grain to yield one pound of animal flesh is based on the assumption that to yield animal flesh, one needs to first grow and harvest grain.

This simply isn't the case. Yes, this is how our industrial food supply has been organized, and yes, this is how animals grown in feedlots are raised. However, many of the animals we're now feeding grain are not biologically designed to digest it. Ruminants—cows, sheep, and goats—have multiple stomachs specifically for the breakdown of cellulose in grass. Allowing the animals full access to pasture allows them to convert biomass indigestible by humans (grass) into what we can digest (protein and fat). Feeding cows a predominantly grain-based diet is not only inefficient and destructive environmentally, it's also harmful to the animal. Cows fed grain develop *acidosis* (excessive acid) in their stomachs, a health concern to both the animals and to us, as this highly acid environment is a breeding ground for a particularly resistant strain of *E. coli* that isn't found in grass-fed cattle (Callaway et al. 2003).

47

So What Meat Can We Eat?

Now that we've looked at the issues concerning meat consumption, let's translate this into the practical. What's the responsible way to eat meat?

Quality Over Quantity

The typical American is most certainly not protein deficient. In fact, quite the opposite. In her book *What to Eat* (2006), Marion Nestle shares that "today, the per capita annual share of meat available for consumption in the United States is about 102 pounds of chicken, 98 pounds of beef, 67 pounds of pork, 17 pounds of turkey, and 2 or 3 pounds of lamb and veal" (Nestle 2006, 141). We certainly don't need to be eating *more* meat. Our demand for quantity at the expense of quality has been a key factor in the quest to raise animals for slaughter faster and at lower cost. Meeting this demand is what directly led to the development of confinement operations, grain feeding, and ultimately many of the environmental, health, and animal-welfare challenges I've described.

If you choose to consume meat, then my recommendation to you would be to eat higher quality meat and eat less of it. A small portion of meat—say, three to four ounces—with one meal daily, or even every other day if you find that works for you, is sufficient (unless perhaps you're an athlete and protein needs to be a more significant part of your daily diet). Depending on how much meat you currently consume, this could actually reduce the amount you spend on meat while vastly increasing the quality. So splurge on the good stuff and just eat it sparingly.

Pasture Perfect

As you may have guessed by now, the best meat to eat is that from animals that were raised in a more naturally suitable environment. This means cattle out in pasture eating grass and occasionally seeds (when grasses are seeding naturally and seasonally), chickens pecking at dirt and grubs, and pigs allowed to roam and forage for anything they can find.

Your next question, as mine was, is probably "How on earth do I find meat from such animals?" Here's a basic guide to the different labels and classifications of meats.

Grass Fed or Grass Finished

Ruminants—cows, sheep, goats, and buffalo—are described as grass fed or grass finished. The USDA has not yet come to a formal definition of either grass fed or grass finished, but generally speaking, *grass-fed beef* means the cattle ate only grass or forage most of their lives. These animals may have been "finished" on grain, which means they were fed grain in the last 90 to 160 days of their lives. *Grass finished*, on the other hand, is a more specific term meaning that the cattle were fed grass throughout the entire course of their lives, even in the finishing stage (the last 90 to 160 days). Because there is no formal definition, many people use these two terms interchangeably, but ideally you want to find beef that was grass finished.

An important point is that if an animal is grass fed or grass finished, this doesn't necessarily mean it's organic. But it's a rare thing to find a farmer raising grass-fed or grass-finished cattle also using pesticides and growth hormones. Generally speaking, when it comes to ruminants, grass fed or finished is the gold standard in terms of nutritional value, animal welfare, and environmental sustainability.

Pastured

The grass-fed equivalent for pork and poultry is the term *pastured*. As with grass fed and grass finished, the USDA does not yet formally define pastured, but the term is typically used to describe pork and poultry that have been raised on pasture. Both pigs and poultry munch on a variety of things—grasses, to be sure, along with insects in the case of poultry, and just about anything else in the case of not-at-all-picky pigs.

Vegetarian Fed

Sometimes you'll see the label "vegetarian fed" on poultry or eggs. Chickens require full protein and aren't natural vegetarians, which makes this label misleading. Essentially, it means that the chickens weren't fed other ground-up chickens—which is, of course, a very good thing. The challenge with the label is that chickens are natural omnivores; they need protein of some sort. So, if they are truly and exclusively vegetarian fed, this means that they are kept inside their whole lives and receive most of their protein from soy. To me this label indicates a better-than-nothing situation, but I don't actively seek out poultry products labeled "vegetarian fed." Certified organic regulations for poultry and eggs disallow feeding chickens parts of other chickens, so if your meat is organic, this issue has been addressed.

Certified Organic

If meat is certified organic by the USDA, this means that the feed the animals receive is organic. However, "organic" doesn't mean that the animal is either pastured or grass fed. The USDA Certified Organic label means that the animals are fed organic feed and aren't treated with antibiotics or growth hormones. It also means there were no genetically modified ingredients in their feed and that the resulting meat isn't irradiated. As of 2010, the certification does have some minimal pasturing requirements, but for the most part, the bulk of the animals' diet is still grain, albeit organic grain.

One of the really nice things about eating meat that is certified organic is that you know the farm it came from was inspected by an independent third party not affiliated with the farm. Therefore, you can be assured that the meat you're eating is meeting these standards.

Free Range and Cage Free

The term *free range* applies to poultry and means that the chickens or turkeys have access to the outdoors. According to the USDA website, free range means that "producers must demonstrate to the Agency that the poultry has been allowed access to the outside" (U. S. Department of Agriculture 2010). They are not required to have access to actual pasture; "free range" simply means access to the outdoors. In other words, a little concrete outdoor area is sufficient. There are no specifications for when the animals get outside or for how long. In fact, you can't even be sure that they actually made it to the outside area provided. In many cases, free range means that there is a small door at the end of a barn that the birds can go through to get outside if they choose. If there's nothing out there for them—no dirt, no grubs, no grasses, no shelter—the chance that they actually go out is slim.

While free-range is a term that is legally defined by the USDA, "cage free" is not formally defined. *Cage free* typically means that the birds aren't kept in wildly overcrowded, stacked cages. It doesn't mean that they are roaming about freely outdoors, or even that they have access to the outdoors, and it doesn't say anything about how many birds are together. It simply means that they aren't kept in cages.

Natural

In my mind, this is the most ridiculous of all labels on meat. Technically speaking, any and all fresh meat is "natural." In the industry, it simply means that the meat contains no artificial colors, it has been "minimally processed," and there are no additional, artificial ingredients. It says nothing about how the animal was raised, what it ate, or the conditions it was kept in. If meat isn't even "natural," then my advice is to run to the nearest exit.

In Summary

Naked meat is meat that comes from animals raised traditionally, healthfully, and sustainably. It's meat that you can feel really good about eating and is well worth searching out. Perhaps the biggest challenge pertaining to naked meat is finding it. We'll examine shopping issues more thoroughly in chapter 12, "Shop Naked," and I'll include even more information on my website: www.eatnakednow.com

If you're a meat eater, take an inventory of what meat you eat most frequently and try to find a more naked version. Yes, it might be a little more expensive than what you're currently eating, but serve smaller portions and go for the higher quality. If you don't eat meat now but are curious to try, pick a type of meat that appeals to you and find the most naked source possible. Start small, try it out, and see how your body responds. Ultimately, your body will be your best guide.

Meat: Good, Better, Best		
	Poultry and Pork	**Ruminants**
Best	Pastured	Grass-finished or grass-fed
Next best	Organic	Organic
Okay	Free range	
Steer clear	"Natural" or other	"Natural" or other

6

naked dairy and eggs

One thing I could never give up in my vegetarian days—preventing me from ever being truly vegan—was cheese. I love me some cheese. I always have, and I imagine I always will. I have yet to find a cheese I don't like, except perhaps some of the cheese "products" that taste more like petroleum than anything else and bear no resemblance to the real thing. What I didn't give much consideration to in those days was the fact that the cheese I loved so dearly was coming from animals living in conditions quite similar to—in some cases worse than—those that prompted me to stop eating meat. Certainly I wasn't killing the animals in order to benefit from their protein, but that didn't mean that they were living happy, healthy, contented lives. In many cases, the exact opposite was true.

There is something very emotional about dairy products. They're deeply nourishing in a way that's perhaps reminiscent of mother's milk. For some, it really can be the ultimate comfort food. And then to others, it's completely repulsive, and the idea of drinking the milk that is really intended for that animal's own young is stomach turning.

Emotional attachment aside, many of the issues and considerations pertaining to dairy and eggs are similar to those in chapter 5. As with meat, the choice to consume dairy and eggs is an extremely personal one.

Dairy products are among the top five allergens, so there are certainly many people who can't tolerate them. Only you and your body know what works best for you. As in chapter 5, my goal with this one is not to convince you to eat or not eat dairy and eggs. My intent is to shed light on the issues pertaining to these foods so that you can make conscious decisions that promote your health, help sustain the environment, and protect the welfare of the animals that produce these foods.

Milk: Perfect Food or Poison?

The question of whether milk and dairy products are healthy or harmful is hotly debated in the nutrition field. Fierce dairy advocates argue that it's the perfect food: it's an optimal whole food, with the ideal balance of protein, fat, and carbohydrates, and it contains good amounts of vital nutrients such as vitamins A and D, and calcium. And then there are the fierce dairy opponents who come equipped with a long list of health ailments linked to dairy consumption: allergies, asthma, certain cancers, digestive issues, and even heart disease, to name a few. Who's right and who's wrong? Well, it's not that simple.

All Milk Is Not Created Equal

It would be so convenient to be able to discuss milk and dairy products generally in one big category, but this would be inaccurate. Milk comes in a variety of qualities. There is the milk that comes from cows raised mostly outdoors on grass without growth hormones. This product has a very different nutritional profile than the milk that comes from cows raised mostly indoors on corn and soy with growth hormones to boost milk production and antibiotics to treat the ailments that result from overmilking and dirty, crowded conditions. Just as with the meat from a cow raised on grass, dairy from grass-fed cows has more of the anti-inflammatory omega-3 fatty acids, vitamin A, beta-carotene, and the omega-6 fatty acid CLA, which I introduced in the previous chapter. This kind of milk is also free of *recombinant bovine growth hormone* (rBGH), a synthetic growth hormone banned from use in Canada and Europe for its suspected link to cancer. Milk in the United States that is produced in industrial milk operations is from cows that have been treated with rBGH. So, unless your milk is organic or labeled to indicate that it is rBGH free, you're drinking milk produced with this hormone. Industrially produced milk also has far lower (if any) levels of CLA and significantly reduced amounts of the other nutrients I've mentioned.

So, as a first consideration, we need to determine the living conditions and diet of the animal. In chapter 5 we examined the environmental sustainability and animal-welfare considerations of industrial meat production. Just as with meat, there are more nutritional benefits available from milk produced by animals that have been raised in their natural environment.

The Great Debate: Pasteurized or Raw?

Things get really hot and heavy in the discussion about dairy when we talk about pasteurized versus raw milk. *Pasteurization* is the process of briefly heating milk in order to kill harmful pathogens and bacteria. Originally developed in the 1800s by Louis Pasteur, the technique was designed to mitigate serious illness and death from milk contaminated by disease-causing pathogens. At the time, unsanitary conditions, lack of refrigeration, and slow transportation made such a measure necessary and appropriate. Today, with vastly improved sanitary conditions, refrigerated steel vats for milk storage, and much speedier transportation options, it would seem that raw milk is again a viable option. There is a whole contingent of raw-milk advocates who argue that pasteurization is no longer necessary or appropriate in certain conditions—namely, in highly sanitary dairies where the animals are raised in natural settings (mostly outdoors on pasture), fed

---

A NOTE ABOUT GOAT'S AND SHEEP'S MILK

For several reasons, goat's milk and sheep's milk are often recommended as alternatives to cow's milk. For one, most goats and sheep are pastured and aren't given the same levels of hormones and antibiotics as used in large dairy operations. This means the milk is cleaner. For another, the proteins in goat's and sheep's milk appear to be more easily digested by humans than the proteins in cow's milk. Therefore, people with dairy allergies are sometimes able to tolerate these milks more easily than they can cow's milk. If you're not able to tolerate cow's milk (including raw milk, as we'll discuss in a moment), try goat's or sheep's milk and see how your body responds.

---

what they're biologically designed to eat (grass), and not pumped full of growth hormones or antibiotics.

Yet, if pasteurization kills harmful bacteria, then why would anyone challenge its necessity? The trouble with pasteurization is that it can undermine the quality of the milk. Not only does pasteurization kill bad bacteria and pathogens, it also kills or severely damages some of the most important nutrients in the milk, nutrients that make milk the whole, nutrient-dense superfood that its proponents claim it to be.

Lactase and Lactose Intolerance

Pasteurization damages the delicate enzyme *lactase*, which is required to digest the milk sugar *lactose*. As babies, all of us produce lactase. That's how we're able to digest breast milk. But in some people, lactase production declines massively by around age four, when, being fully weaned, we would have no more need for it. When drinking raw milk, this doesn't pose a problem: the milk comes with its own lactase to digest the lactose. The problem occurs when drinking pasteurized milk. Having no lactase in either the milk or the person drinking it leads to digestive distress and diarrhea, a condition called *lactose intolerance*. And yet, many people who are lactose intolerant not only tolerate raw milk but thrive on it.

Beneficial Bacteria and Immunity

Along with the harmful bacteria, pasteurization also kills the beneficial bacteria in milk. Heat is not selective. Anything present in the milk that can be damaged by heat is damaged, which means the good bacteria as well as the bad. Beneficial bacteria are fundamental to a healthy digestive tract and strong immune system, both of which are compromised in its absence. Pasteurized milk doesn't contain these beneficial bacteria, although some good bacteria can be regained by culturing the milk into such foods as yogurt or kefir.

Important Vitamins

Pasteurization destroys or greatly reduces vitamins A, B$_{12}$, C, and D (Fallon 2001). Food manufacturers replace the vitamin D with synthetic vitamin D because, without it, your body can't access the calcium in the milk. But many question the nutritional value of a synthetic vitamin rather than one that occurs naturally, and the other damaged vitamins aren't replaced.

When Pasteurization Is Necessary

Learning about all the nutrients that pasteurization damages and understanding that there is a safe way to consume raw milk might lead you to wonder, as I did, why pasteurization is a federally regulated requirement. Why is raw milk not only so difficult to procure, but illegal in some states? The answer to this question can become heated and political in a hurry, and unfortunately we don't have the room to go into the debate here. If you're interested in this topic, I've included a few starting points on my website: www.eatnakednow.com.

For now, pasteurization is necessary and mandated appropriately when it comes to industrial dairy production, where harmful pathogens and bacteria are abundant. We know that the health of the cow is compromised when we take it off pasture and bring it into a confinement feedlot operation. It hurts the cow, reduces the nutritional value of the milk, and increases the likelihood of harmful bacteria and pathogens being in the milk.

From a shelf-life and distribution perspective, pasteurization is also favorable. It extends shelf-life to two to three weeks. In the case of UHT (*ultra-high-temperature pasteurization*, in which milk is heated briefly to 280 degrees Fahrenheit and then stored in aseptic boxes), milk stays "fresh" for months. Commercially, this is appealing.

Would I recommend consuming raw dairy products that come from industrially produced milk? Absolutely not. However, a better question might be, would I recommend consuming *any* dairy product that comes from industrially produced milk? No. The poor quality of the milk, of the environment the animals live in, and of the diet they eat far outweigh any health benefits that consuming such products could confer. And these are the very things that make pasteurization the only safe way to consume the milk. As Mark McAfee, CEO of Organic Pastures Dairy, writes, "Pasteurization does not create clean milk; it just kills filthy milk" (McAfee 2010, 82).

If you'd like to try raw milk, I encourage you to become familiar with the safety considerations. An excellent resource is found in the chapter "The Safety of Raw versus Pasteurized Milk" in Ron Schmid's book *The Untold Story of Milk* (2003). Ultimately, it's impossible to guarantee the safety of any food, raw or pasteurized. Pasteurization doesn't guarantee safety, as contamination can and does happen after milk is pasteurized. When looking for a safe source of raw milk, look for a dairy that feeds its cows grass and has a reputation for high quality. If you're in a state such as California that allows the retail sale of raw milk, look for dairies with certified raw milk. Some dairies, such as Organic Pastures, post results of inspections and laboratory analysis of their milk on a regular basis. If you have seriously compromised immunity or are taking immunosuppressive drugs, be particularly diligent about your source of raw milk, or consider skipping dairy altogether.

What About Organic?

As with organic meat, dairy products that are certified organic by the USDA are from cows fed exclusively organic feed, that are not given any synthetic growth hormones, and that have some access to pasture. This doesn't mean that they are fed exclusively grass, are spending most of their time outdoors on pasture, or are treated humanely, or that the milk that comes from them is safe enough to be sold raw. Most certified organic milk is pasteurized.

Would I recommend consuming pasteurized dairy products from these animals? My answer is a cautious yes, but use only those products that have been cultured, such as yogurt, kefir, or cheese. The culturing process replaces some of the beneficial bacteria, and the lactose is largely pre-digested by the cultures, helping you to avoid the digestive difficulties the uncultured milk may cause.

Other Considerations for Dairy

Beyond the decisions about pasteurization and whether to choose organic, there are other issues to investigate when determining which dairy products to include in your diet.

Homogenized or Not?

Before studying nutrition, I never even considered whether milk was homogenized or not. I didn't really have an idea what homogenization was.

To me, homogenized meant whole. I remember my grandmother drinking "homogenized" milk—a thick, creamy, and (in my eyes) gross beverage. Because it wasn't the 2 percent or skim that we had at our house, I assumed (incorrectly) that homogenized meant full fat.

When milk is whole, the cream naturally settles to the top. *Homogenization* is the process by which the cream and the milk are forcibly combined so that they don't separate when left standing. There are two reasons for milk producers to homogenize milk. For one, it ensures that the cream (what used to be the most valued part of the milk) is distributed evenly throughout so that every bottle has the same amount. Another, much less appetizing reason for homogenizing milk is directly related to pasteurization. Author Nina Planck describes it best: "After pasteurization, dead white blood cells and bacteria form a sludge that sinks to the bottom of the milk. Homogenization spreads this unsightly mass throughout the milk and makes it disappear" (Planck 2006, 76). Yum. This is one of the reasons why I don't like to drink pasteurized milk. The harmful bacteria might be dead, but their carcasses are still in the milk. Since I'm the squeamish type, that thought doesn't particularly appeal to me.

Whole or Skim?

I was raised on 2 percent milk, and in my nonfat days I taught myself to drink the pale, rather flavorless skim. When I was a little girl, my grandmother's whole milk tasted far too rich and creamy for me, and I couldn't drink the big glasses I was accustomed to drinking at home. As it turns out, that fat is really important.

Taking the fat out of the milk makes it difficult for your body to access and use two very important vitamins found in the milk: vitamin A and D, both of which are fat soluble (meaning that they need fat to be absorbed and used by your body). Without the vitamin D, in particular, the calcium in the milk is not as absorbable by your body. As a result, reduced-fat milk always has synthetic vitamins A and D added to it, with debatable health benefits.

The other challenge with reduced-fat milk is that it's often fortified with powdered milk for added protein. Unfortunately, powdered milk contains oxidized (damaged) cholesterol, which is highly damaging to arterial walls (Reaven et al. 1991), far more so than undamaged cholesterol. (We'll take a closer look at cholesterol in chapter 8, "Naked Fats.") Unfortunately, milk producers aren't required to include powdered milk on the ingredient list, so there's no way of knowing whether it's included or not.

These days, I prefer whole milk. I certainly don't drink the volumes I used to when I was young, but I now love the rich, creamy taste, and shaking up the bottle to mix up the cream with the rest of the milk always delights me. As for the fat content, I'm a big fan of healthy, real fats, and whole milk has a good amount of them. See chapter 8 for an in-depth examination of what I mean by "healthy" when it comes to fat.

Milk Substitutes

Let's say you're not able to find raw milk from grass-fed cows in your area, or you're allergic to the casein (protein) in the milk. A wander down the milk aisle in your local grocery store will present you with a plethora of nondairy milk substitutes: soy milks of all varieties and flavors, rice milk, almond milk, coconut milk…the choices seem endless.

None of these are truly a naked food. All of them have been processed, many have been sweetened (even if using natural sweeteners), and none come close to reproducing the nutritional value of real milk. If pressed, I'd go with unsweetened almond milk or unsweetened coconut milk, but neither would be a regular part of my diet. Avoid soy milk in particular, as it is an unfermented and highly processed soy product that will be incredibly hard on your digestive system. For more about soy and the health issues related to it, see chapter 2, "If You're Not Eating Naked, What Are You Eating?"

MILK: ONLY FOR BABY COWS?

A common argument against dairy consumption is that cow's milk is for baby cows, not humans. Yes, fundamentally this is true. However, there is no nutrient in the milk that isn't appropriate for the human diet. While I can understand where this argument is going, no food is really designed "for" human consumption. As Nina Planck aptly puts it, "After all, the tomato was designed to make more tomato plants, not pasta sauce" (2006, 56).

Milk: To Drink or Not to Drink?

Truly naked dairy is raw, whole, and unhomogenized and comes from cows that have been raised on pasture and grass, without growth hormones or antibiotics. The moment you pasteurize milk, homogenize milk, or remove any of its fat content, it's no longer a naked food. As Marion Nestle writes, "[Conventional] milk is now a processed food, routinely clarified, separated, reconstituted, homogenized, and pasteurized—a big change from the way things used to be" (2006, 91).

As I've said, the decision about whether or not to consume dairy and then which dairy to consume is entirely yours. My clients and others often ask what decisions I've made about milk, given all these considerations. The issues can certainly be overwhelming.

Do I drink milk and consume dairy products? Absolutely. I'm not a big milk drinker, but when I do, I only drink milk that's raw, whole, and unhomogenized, and that comes from a clean, reputable dairy with healthy, grass-fed cows. This is a slightly easier task for me in California, where dairy farmers can sell raw milk through retail stores. If you're not lucky enough to live in a state where raw milk is as easily found, you can still hunt it down, but it takes some effort. I've included resources on my website to get you started: www.eatnakednow.com.

If you're not comfortable with the risks involved in drinking raw milk (and that is entirely your choice to make), then choose those dairy products that have been cultured, like yogurt, kefir, cheese, or buttermilk. Culturing dairy will bring back some of the nutrition lost during pasteurization and also make it more digestible, so this is a good "next-best" scenario. As I confessed earlier in the chapter, I am a cheese lover and I always seek out whole, raw-milk cheeses. If these aren't available, I'll settle for organic, but I will never consume conventional or the rubbery low-fat varieties. I'm much the same with yogurt: I look for raw-milk yogurt, but if I can't get it, I'll settle for whole, unflavored, organic yogurt.

A Little About Eggs

The issues pertaining to eggs mirror most of the issues pertaining to chickens. As with the meat that comes from the chicken, the most nutritious eggs are those that come from pastured chickens allowed to peck and roam around in the dirt, eating a mix of grain, grubs, grasses, and other forage.

These eggs are also the best choice from the environmental and animal-welfare perspectives as well. There are a few specific considerations that pertain only to eggs, however, so let's address those here.

Yolks, Whites, or Whole?

In her book *Real Foods: What to Eat and Why* (2006), Nina Planck opens up her discussion on eggs with a section entitled "The Abominable Egg-White Omelet." I love this title, as it perfectly captures my feelings about this topic. Whole eggs or, more specifically, egg yolks, were the unfortunate victims of the anticholesterol sentiments that have dominated the nutrition field over the last forty years. Even with multiple respected studies clearly vindicating the highly nutritious yolk, the fear created around consuming it runs strong and deep (Hu et al. 1999; Kritchevsky and Kritchevsky 2000). I spend a lot of time with my nutrition clients explaining to them why it's not only okay but preferable to eat the whole egg. Usually this news is met with a mixture of disbelief and delight.

A whole egg is one of nature's most perfect foods, and it comes jam-packed with nutrients. It's an excellent source of protein, important fatty acids, antioxidants, lecithin, vitamins A, B, E, and D, and folic acid. To many people's surprise, the yolk is actually the most nutritionally dense part of the egg, as it's the source of the fatty acids, important antioxidants, vitamins, and, yes, the cholesterol. As we'll discuss in more detail in chapter 8, cholesterol is actually an important part of our diet, and it is not the consumption of cholesterol itself that's responsible for hardening our arteries and causing heart disease.

Omega-3 Enriched

One of the labels you'll see on an egg carton is the description "omega-3 enriched." What does this mean? Omega-3 fatty acids are important, anti-inflammatory fatty acids that are at chronically low levels in the North American diet. You'll find the greatest amount of these fatty acids in eggs from chickens that have been pastured. Pastured chickens also produce eggs with the optimal one-to-one ratio of omega-3 and omega-6 fatty acids (one unit of omega-3 to one unit of omega-6). On the other hand, industrially produced eggs have an imbalanced one-to-twenty ratio of omega-3 to omega-6 fatty acids. (See chapter 8, "Naked Fats," for a more in-depth look at the two omega essential fatty acids.)

To rectify this imbalance and increase the amount of omega-3 fatty acids in their eggs, some farmers add flaxseed to the chickens' feed if they're not going to be pastured. That's what the label "omega-3 enriched" means. If you're not able to find pastured eggs, organic, omega-3-enhanced eggs are a good next-best option.

Extra Large

A special consideration for eggs is their size. When you see the labels "extra-large" or "jumbo," it's possible that these eggs are from chickens that were forced to molt by being deprived of food for several days. Unfortunately, this is common practice in the industry as a way to extend the egg-producing life of the hen. When hens that have been force-molted start to lay again, they lay fewer but larger eggs. Some egg producers are investigating non-feed-deprivation means of speeding up the molting process, but there's no way to know unless you talk directly to the producer. If you're buying your eggs from a farmers' market or small producer, ask them if they molt their hens or if they let the hens go out of lay for part of the year (a natural part of the laying cycle for the hen).

The Great Egg Hunt

One of the most challenging things about sourcing eggs is finding those that have come from chickens truly allowed to live a "chicken" life with real access to the outdoors, living vegetation, natural light, and dust baths. As we discussed in chapter 5, the definitions of cage free and free range are so broad they are almost meaningless. There's quite a range in quality of egg and treatment of the chickens within these labels. A helpful tool in finding pastured eggs is the Cornucopia Institute's Organic Egg Scorecard (http://www.cornucopia.org/organic-egg-scorecard/).

In Summary

The conversation about naked eggs is a fairly simple one: find eggs from chickens that are raised in an environment appropriate to the bird's natural needs, and you'll get the most nutritional benefit while ensuring the welfare of the chickens. See the table below for the eggs to look for and those to avoid.

Naked dairy, on the other hand, is a lot more confusing. Raw, whole, unhomogenized milk and milk products that come from a clean dairy that raises its cows on grass are ideal—and yet incredibly difficult to find. If it must be pasteurized, then whole, organic, and unhomogenized milk is next best; but again, is still quite difficult to find, and many people aren't able to digest it. I strongly recommend limiting your intake of milk that's pasteurized unless it's been cultured (cheese, yogurt, kefir, or buttermilk). Of course, another option is to try goat's milk or sheep's milk and see how your body likes those.

Dairy and Eggs: Good, Better, Best

	Milk	Other Dairy Products (Cheese, Yogurt)	Eggs
Best	Grass fed, raw, unhomogenized	Made from raw milk from grass-fed cows	From pastured chickens
Next best	Organic, pasteurized, unhomogenized	Made from organic, pasteurized milk	Organic, omega-3 enhanced or not
Okay	Organic, pasteurized cow's milk Unsweetened almond milk Unsweetened coconut milk	Made from conventional whole milk, unflavored and unsweetened	From free-range chickens
Steer clear	Conventional, lowfat or nonfat, or flavored cow's milk Milk substitutes	Made from conventional, low-fat or nonfat milk, sweetened, or flavored Made from milk substitutes	Extra-large or jumbo eggs "Natural" or other factory-farmed eggs Egg substitutes Liquid eggs Powdered eggs

7
naked fish

I've always eaten fish and loved it. When I was little, my mom called it brain food and we ate it often, but always in the same ways. My understanding of fish was limited to tuna sandwiches and creamed salmon on rice (which is actually quite delicious). I'm not exactly sure when I realized that the fish we ate at home didn't just come out of a can and once lived in water. It's not something I gave a lot of thought to. I even forgot to include fish in the early drafts of this book. Funny, since I eat it at least once or twice a week.

Fish Quandaries

Nutritionally speaking, the topic of fish and seafood is incredibly confusing. Fish is touted as vitally important nutritionally, but also often characterized as a toxic storehouse. Choosing fish wisely is anything but straightforward, with seemingly endless issues to consider. Is the fish farmed or wild? Where it is on the food chain? What waters did it come from? How was it fished? What did it eat? And how well stocked or depleted is the fishery for that type of fish? I don't know about you, but that's far more information than my brain can handle at any given point in time.

To complicate the issue, no one can agree on how much fish you should consume or how often. The Food and Drug Administration, the Environmental Protection Agency, the Environmental Working Group, and various fish-industry groups all give completely different recommendations. Whom to believe?

Interestingly, this is the area of meat consumption into which some vegetarians first dip their toes. The term for this is officially a *pescetarian*, essentially a vegetarian who also eats fish. Considering the incredible complexities of the issues pertaining to fish, I've always wondered about this. Maybe it's because we're further removed from fish and don't identify with them as much as we do land animals. More likely, it's because we've heard that they're jam-packed with nutrients and are keen to get our nutritional needs met.

Let's take a look at the issues, starting with why fish is so good for you.

Health Benefits of Consuming Fish

Fish is the best and only direct source of the omega-3 fatty acids EPA (eicosapentaenoic acid) and DHA (docosahexaenoic acid). The body can make these two fatty acids from ALA (alpha-linolenic acid), which is found in walnuts and flaxseeds, but it does so inefficiently. The process by which your body does this conversion requires vitamins and minerals that are often depleted (vitamin B_6, magnesium, calcium, and zinc), and this process can easily be interrupted by such common things as excess insulin and the consumption of trans-fatty acids, aspirin, alcohol, and NSAIDS (nonsteroidal anti-inflammatory drugs, such as ibuprofen and naproxen).

EPA and DHA are very important fatty acids for several reasons. They're vital to the development of the brain, which is mostly (60 percent) fat, much of which is DHA (Muskiet et al. 2004). That's significant. As we'll see in chapter 8, "Naked Fats," omega-3 fats play a significant role in bringing down inflammation, which is one of the reasons they're often prescribed by doctors for patients who are showing early warning signs of being at risk for heart disease. EPA and DHA specifically have been shown to reduce levels of triglycerides and VLDL (very low-density lipoprotein), a harmful type of cholesterol (McKenney and Sica 2007; Kinsella 1987). They have also been indicated in aiding in the prevention of certain types of cancer (De Deckere 1999), strengthening the immune system

(Damsgaard et al. 2007), and alleviating depression (Mischoulon et al. 2009).

And it's not just about the fatty acids. Fish and seafood are also excellent sources of protein, the fat-soluble vitamins A and D, and important minerals such as calcium, phosphorous, iodine, and zinc. With as impressive a list of health benefits as this, it's clear why fish has a reputation as a nutritionally dense and healthful food. So, what are the issues we need to be concerned about?

Health Concerns with Fish Consumption

Much like the concerns around meat, the challenges pertaining to fish consumption deal with the quality of the fish, which is directly related to the quality of the environment the fish was living in and what it ate. But there are also certain concerns that are specific to fish, namely the contamination by two toxins: methylmercury and PCBs (polychlorinated biphenyls).

Fish: A Toxic Storehouse?

The issue most often raised when it comes to fish consumption is that of the levels of methylmercury and PCBs found in the fish flesh (where methylmercury is stored) and fat (where PCBs accumulate).

Methylmercury is mercury (in water) that has been methylated by microorganisms (a complex series of processes that transforms mercury into its methylated, and most toxic, form), making it incredibly easy for humans to absorb. It's the most dangerous form of mercury for human health, and we are exposed to it by eating large, carnivorous fish. These bigger fish eat smaller fish that eat diets of methylmercury-stuffed plankton in infected waterways. Methylmercury is most dangerous for pregnant women, as it crosses the placenta and enters the fetus's brain, where it wreaks havoc. This is why doctors recommend that pregnant women be very careful with their consumption of tuna, a large carnivorous fish that often has high levels of this contaminant.

When it comes to PCBs, or polychlorinated biphenyls, the story gets uglier. All fish, small and large, regardless of where they are on the food chain, have some degree of PCB contamination. PCBs have been shown to damage human reproduction and development, alter immune function, and create problems with the skin (Aoki 2001). PCBs get into our waterways from pesticides (another good reason to eat organic) and other industrial wastes and emissions. Even those that have been banned from use (DDT is a well-known example) persist in the environment for years. While all fish contain some amounts of PCBs, contamination levels increase as you move up the food chain, much like they do with methylmercury contamination. Also, fish that come from fish farms have significantly higher levels of PCBs.

The problem with both of these toxins isn't about the fish itself. It's the issue of industrial waste getting into waterways, where it is then absorbed and consumed by the fish in increasing levels of contamination as you go up the food chain.

Addressing These Concerns

While it's impossible to know the toxicity of any given fish without testing that specific fish, you can minimize your exposure to these two toxins by avoiding large, carnivorous fish such as swordfish, shark, king mackerel, and albacore tuna, and instead favoring smaller fish lower on the food chain such as anchovy, herring, trout, and tilapia. This strategy is most important for women of childbearing age, those planning to be or already pregnant, women who are breastfeeding, and small children.

Wild Fish or Overfished?

The debate of wild versus farmed fish is the next point of contention. My knee-jerk reaction, I'll confess, is to immediately prioritize wild. After all, "wild" indicates that the fish is living in its natural environment, eating what it is biologically designed and inclined to eat, and presumably living a happy, if interrupted, fish life. In my mind, it's the aquatic equivalent to grass-fed beef.

The nutritional profile of wild fish versus farmed fish confirms my instinct. Studies have shown that farmed salmon, for example, have significantly higher levels of PCBs and other toxins than wild salmon (Foran et al. 2005) and that wild fish have a higher percent of omega-3 fatty acids (Ferreira et al. 2010). This seems simple enough. Can't we eat wild fish and leave it at that?

A NOTE ABOUT SURIMI

Surimi is the fake crab or other seafood that you find most commonly in California rolls at sushi restaurants. It's the contemporary and industrialized version of a traditional preservation method used by the Japanese for some nine hundred years. It is among the most processed foods I know.

Marian Nestle describes the modern-day version of this technique in *What to Eat*: "They wash the flesh of the fish repeatedly until it loses all odor and color; drain it; add cornstarch, other binders, sugar, flavors, and maybe even real fish; shape it into blocks; form it into a paste that they can shape and paint to look like whatever they want it to be; and freeze it. That is surimi" (2006, 223).

Wow. There's nothing naked about that. Avoid it.

Unfortunately, no. One of the most pressing issues concerning fish is overfishing, which leads to dwindling fish stocks. *Overfishing* is what it sounds like: fishing at a greater rate than the fish can reproduce, which means that, over time, whole species can be brought to the brink of extinction. A recent example of this phenomenon was the Atlantic cod fishery, which was severely overfished in the 1970s and 1980s, ultimately leading to a complete collapse of the fishery in the early 1990s. This is devastating not only to the fish but also to the local economies and fishermen who depend on this resource for their livelihood.

A quick perusal of environmental organizations dealing with issues pertaining to wild fish stocks is discouraging. According to a report by the Food and Agriculture Organization of the United Nations, more than 70 percent of the world's fisheries are fully exploited, overexploited, or significantly depleted (2005, 6). This isn't something to be ignored, as our collective appetite for fish is anything but declining. What is the solution? Enter candidate number one: the fish farm.

Fish Farms: Feedlots of the Sea?

With stocks of wild fish dwindling, our global consumption of fish is increasing (World Health Organization 2002) and we have ever more recommendations from nutrition professionals to increase our fish consumption. In this context, the proposed and seemingly logical solution has been aquaculture—fish farms—where we breed and grow fish in "controlled" environments.

My gut reaction to the fish farm is similar to my reaction to a feedlot. It's no surprise that many of the issues in water farm operations mirror those on land. Fish pellets used as feed are certainly no match for the fish's natural diet. This deficiency impacts the nutritional profile of the fish and creates other less-than-appetizing side effects. For instance, salmon farmers add dyes to the fish feed so that the flesh is the nice pink we expect to see in salmon. Without this dye, farmed salmon is gray, since the pellets they're fed in captivity don't contain krill, which is responsible for the deep and beautiful pink color we all associate with salmon. Would you eat gray salmon? Me neither. Enough said.

Overcrowded fish pens cause significant environmental damage to marine environments, not to mention an unpleasant situation for the fish. Because overcrowded conditions tend to foster illness and concentrated filth, there is a widespread use of pesticides, disinfectants, and antibiotics. These additives, along with tremendous amounts of fish waste, end up polluting local waters (Goldburg, Elliott, and Naylor 2001). Fish are difficult to contain and often escape. These fish then compete with wild local species for food and sometimes even crossbreed with wild fish, which further damages the local fishery.

If wild fish stocks are mostly overfished and fish farming isn't a viable solution, what does this mean for our fish-rich diets?

Navigating Through the Issues

Marian Nestle put it best:

> To make an intelligent choice of fish at a supermarket, you have to know more than you can possibly imagine about nutrition, fish toxicology, and the life cycle and ecology of fish—what kind of fish it is, what it eats, where it was caught, and whether it was farmed or wild. If you are at all concerned about environmental issues, you will also want to know how it was caught and raised and whether its stocks are sustainable (2006, 182–3).

I get exhausted just thinking about it.

The situation isn't quite as desperate a picture as I've painted. For one, there *are* well-managed wild fisheries. The Alaskan wild salmon fishery is one example of this. And there are also certain fish—mostly herbivores such as carp, catfish, and tilapia, and mollusks such as oysters and mussels—that do well in aquaculture environments. This is true provided the environment is clean, the species appropriately chosen, and the farm managed in a sustainable manner. The challenge is determining which is which and staying on top of all the pertinent information needed to make a good choice.

Fortunately for all of us, there are people and organizations that are up-to-date on all of the issues, and they have kindly shared that information in what is called a "fish list." This is a pocket guide that you can carry with you that tells you which fish you can enjoy safely, which fish to consume in moderation, and which to avoid completely. Because this information changes regularly, is different from region to region, and is constantly being updated, I'm not going to include my "Good, Better, Best" table here. Instead I'm going to point you to the best list that currently exists, developed by the Monterey Bay Aquarium and its Seafood Watch program. Go to www.seafoodwatch.org to download a current list specific to your region that lets you know what fish is okay to enjoy, which you need to be cautious with, and which you should just avoid altogether.

EAT NAKED ON A BUDGET

You won't often find me suggesting canned food over fresh, but in the case of fish, it can be a simple and affordable solution. Wild canned salmon is quite widely available, and much more affordable than fresh. A can of sardines is an excellent to-go snack. I know, that sounds just plain weird, but consider that sardines are a great protein hit from a small fish low on the food chain, jam-packed with those good fats.

In Summary

Fish is packed with a nutritional punch, but it's important to find fish that's truly naked, not always an easy task. Generally speaking, wild is preferable, but farmed fish, particularly small fish like tilapia, catfish, and carp, can be farmed safely. Your best bet is to download a fish list from a trustworthy source and use that as your guide. If the topic of fish floats your boat, I've included more resources on my website: www.eatnakednow.com.

8
naked fats

Fat is good for you. Not only is it good for you, it's an absolutely essential part of a healthy diet.

Does this surprise you? It did me. One of the most exciting things I learned about when I first studied nutrition was the important role of fats in our diet. I've already told you that I was a junk-food vegetarian. Did I mention that I was a fat-free junk-food vegetarian? That probably doesn't sound like it's possible, but it was. I ate lots of white pasta, veggies, and low- or no-fat cheese. I couldn't imagine the thought of eating butter. I secretly craved it but thought that if I actually ate it, or any fat for that matter, I might as well apply it directly to my thighs because that's surely where it would go. I went through a phase of not using any oils in my cooking at all. I would sauté my veggies with a little bit of water and use only a squeeze of lemon and no oil on my salads.

I was completely wrong in my demonization of fats, and that was great news. Naturally, I resisted adding fat back into my diet at first. I had been well indoctrinated in the low-fat/no-fat myth, and the idea of eating something that tasted that good and it being *healthy* seemed almost impossible. At best, it was a guilty pleasure; at worst, it was the source of any extra pound or unwanted pimple.

Fats: The Wrongfully Accused

Fats are an incredibly important part of our diet. They are a key source of energy, particularly that nice, steady kind of energy that so many of us long for. Think of energy as a fire: carbohydrates are like the kindling, and fats are like the logs. You would never want to stoke your fire all day on kindling alone. It would burn hot, then die out, burn hot, then die out, and you'd constantly need to be fueling it. Sound like a familiar energy pattern? I see it every day with my clients, and I used to experience this myself all the time. For a good, steady burn, you need some nice big logs. That's exactly what the fat is—the log in your fire that keeps you going between meals and manages your energy levels so they're smooth, gentle, and consistent, not spiking high and then crashing over and over.

Fats are important for more than just their role in energy regulation. As a key component in the makeup of our cell membranes, fats are structurally integral. They're in every single cell in the body. They're responsible for healthy liver function, they play a crucial role in our elimination of toxins, and they are essential for the absorption of the four fat-soluble vitamins: A, D, E, and K. Fats act as a protective lining for our organs. Without fats, we can't use our protein properly. They also play a crucial role in managing inflammation in our bodies, which I'll explain in more depth a little later in this chapter.

Let's not forget that fats make food taste good. When food manufacturers remove fat to make something low-fat or nonfat, the food doesn't taste as good. So, to compensate, they put in sweeteners and artificial flavorings, both of which are harmful to our health. And, appropriately, foods that contain fat usually contain fat-soluble vitamins, which means the fat is required in order to access those vitamins.

Fats also are responsible for triggering our satiation mechanism, which makes us feel full and satisfied at the end of a meal. This is a key reason why nonfat and low-fat diets don't work. If we don't feel satisfied at the end of a meal, we're going to want more—either now or later. There's no amount of willpower that can override this bodily need.

So you can see, fats have been given a bad rap, but they're critical to our health and well-being in many ways. It's unfortunate that this vital macronutrient has the same name as a bodily condition so many of us try to avoid. The consumption of fat in appropriate amounts does not necessarily lead to that bodily condition. Clearly, the elimination of fat from our diets has not succeeded in eliminating body fat. There's got to be more to the story.

Fats 101

To clear up some of the confusion around fats, let me offer you a brief lesson on their biochemistry.

Fatty acids are made up of carbon and hydrogen molecules. There are three types of fatty acids: saturated, monounsaturated, and poly-unsaturated. The basic difference between each of these is the number of carbon atoms with or without two hydrogen atoms bonded to them. Here's the difference.

Saturated fatty acids. In a saturated fatty acid, each carbon atom has bonded with two hydrogen atoms. In other words, it's "saturated" with hydrogen. This saturation makes the fatty acid very stable, which means it can withstand more heat before it becomes rancid. Common examples of saturated fats are butter and coconut oil. An easy way to know if a fat is saturated is if it's solid at room temperature. Saturated fats are ideal for cooking because of their natural ability to withstand heat without being damaged.

Monounsaturated fatty acids. In a monounsaturated fatty acid, one pair of carbon atoms forms a double bond with each other that replaces the bond each would have with one hydrogen atom. So it is unsaturated, but only by one bond. This means the fatty acid is less stable than a satu-rated fatty acid molecule. The classic example of monounsaturated fat is olive oil. The oil in almonds, hazelnuts, and avocados is also monoun-saturated. Monounsaturated fats are liquid at room temperature, but they solidify in the refrigerator. These are okay for cooking, but only at very low temperatures.

Polyunsaturated fatty acids. A polyunsaturated fatty acid has two or more carbon pairs that have bonded together rather than with a hydrogen atom. This means the fatty acid is quite unstable. Examples of polyunsatu-rated fats include most vegetable oils, most seed oils, soybean oil, flaxseed oil, and sunflower oil. These fats are liquid both at room temperature and in the refrigerator, and they should never be used for cooking. This might be surprising, given that so many of our standard cooking oils are exactly these unstable vegetable oils.

There is a fourth type of fatty acid, but I haven't included it in the list above because it's not found in nature. It's the *trans fat*, which is an unsaturated fatty acid that has been either partially or fully hydrogenated.

We took a look at these in chapter 2. To hydrogenate fat, food manufacturers forcibly unpair the carbon double bonds in a polyunsaturated fat and force them to bond with hydrogen atoms. This means they're taking a very unstable fat and artificially making it more stable. In a partially hydrogenated fatty acid, only some carbon molecules have been saturated with hydrogen and carbon-pair bonds remain. In a fully hydrogenated fatty acid, all carbon double bonds have been replaced with hydrogen bonds. This process creates what I call a "Franken-fat," a fat that does not exist in nature and is totally unrecognizable, unusable, and actually quite damaging to the body.

It's All in the Balance

When it comes to our consumption of fats, we need all three of the naturally occurring types of fatty acid in our diet. Every fat contains some of each fatty acid. We call a fat "saturated" if it has more saturated fatty acids than mono- or polyunsaturated fatty acids. While butter has a higher percentage of saturated fatty acids than any other type, it also has both omega-3 and omega-6 fats in it, two essential polyunsaturated fatty acids. The easiest way to get enough of each kind of fat is to use each appropriately: the more stable, saturated fats for cooking at higher temperatures, the less stable, monounsaturated fats for cooking at lower temperatures, and the highly unstable, polyunsaturated fats for things that aren't cooked, for example in salad dressings and unheated sauces.

"Good" Fats vs. "Bad" Fats

We've all heard that there are "good" fats and "bad" fats, and typically it breaks down something like this: good fats are vegetables oils, and bad fats are trans fats, saturated fats, and animal fats (because they're typically higher in saturated fats), with the notable exception of fish oil, which is currently getting lots of kudos for its anti-inflammatory properties. This classification of good and bad fats is inaccurate and misses a critically important factor.

With the notable exception of trans fats (they are indisputably bad), there is no type of fat that is categorically good or bad. What makes it so is the quality of the fat and how it has been processed. Saturated fats are not categorically good or bad. Unsaturated fats are not categorically good or bad. What makes a fat beneficial or harmful to your health is its quality and how it has been extracted from its source. I emphasize this point because it's so different from what most marketing and outdated nutrition wisdom will have us believe. Let's get specific.

Saturated fats have been maligned over the past decades. Accused of increasing heart disease, cancer rates, obesity, and a host of other health challenges, they have been demonized and labeled the primary bad fat. But consider this: saturated fats—in particular, animal fats—have been consumed by humans for thousands of years. In fact, our consumption of animal fats has decreased over the last century, while our consumption of vegetable oils has increased dramatically (Enig 2000). Compare this to the change in the incidence of heart disease, which was rare at the turn of the twentieth century and now, just over a hundred years later, is the leading cause of death. Are saturated animal fats to blame? There is certainly ample research that challenges this link between saturated fats and heart disease (Ravnskov 1998).

Because of the fear of animal fats and saturated fats, vegetable oils have taken over. Unfortunately, being mostly of the mono- and polyunsaturated types, they are quite unstable. Industrial extraction and refinement processes almost always involve heat, which damages these delicate oils, creating free radicals that are extremely damaging to the body. Then they're often stored in clear plastic bottles, which leach chemicals into the oil and allow in light and heat that further damages the oil.

Don't misunderstand me. I'm not saying that we should switch to 100 percent saturated animal fats. It's important to have a balance of all three types of fat, to use them appropriately (for instance, eating unstable vegetable and seed oils cold), and to eat the highest quality we can find.

Quality Is Key

Quality is by far the most important factor in choosing a fat. In this context, quality means a fat that has been extracted and stored in a way that doesn't damage it. This means no hydrogenation or partial hydrogenation and no bleaching or other heat or chemical processes that alter the fat.

A quality vegetable oil is one that has been extracted in a way that doesn't negatively affect the oil and is stored in a way that preserves its nutritional integrity. This means the oil is refrigerated if it's polyunsaturated and stored in a dark glass jar or tin, not in a plastic bottle. And these oils should certainly never be kept right next to or above the stove, where they will be repeatedly subjected to heat.

If the fat is from an animal, quality fat comes from an animal raised in an environment it was biologically designed to live in. For example, butter from grass-fed cows allowed to pasture and move around freely as opposed to butter from grain-fed cows living in a feedlot.

Quality is paramount in fats for several reasons. For one, the nutritional value of a quality fat is superior to a low-quality, refined, or modified version. Take butter that comes from a pastured cow. This butter contains conjugated linoleic acid (CLA), which has anticancer properties, helps prevent weight gain, and stimulates muscle growth. This nutrient is virtually absent in cows fed grain or processed feed (Dhiman et al. 1999). Also, toxins tend to accumulate in fat. This means that if the animal has a high toxic burden from consuming pesticide-laden feed or has received high doses of antibiotics and hormones, that toxic burden is going to be stored in its fat, which we will then eat.

And What About Cholesterol?

You may be thinking, "This is all very well and good, but doesn't eating saturated fat and animal fat generally lead to increased levels of cholesterol?" I'm glad you asked. This is a very important question.

Like saturated fat, cholesterol is another topic that raises alarm bells and sends people running. And, like saturated fat, much of the fear is based on a misunderstanding of cholesterol and its role in the body.

Cholesterol is vitally important to our health. It's used to make all the sex hormones, to use vitamin D properly, and to create bile salts, which are critical for digesting fats and eliminating toxins. It actually (and surprisingly, to many) acts as an antioxidant in the body. And, among its many roles, it is a patching and repair mechanism integral to our body's ability to heal and repair from damage (Enig and Fallon 2006). At the most basic level, what we've come to call "bad" cholesterol, low-density lipoprotein (LDL), is the repair material that is taken to damaged areas. An increase in LDL indicates that there's damage. The "good" cholesterol, high-density lipoprotein (HDL), is the material being removed, which indicates that the repair work is no longer needed. In truth, neither LDL nor HDL is good or bad. Both are important and appropriate responses (Planck 2006).

The conventional approach to managing cholesterol is to measure cholesterol levels and then try to change the levels themselves, rather than looking at what's causing the damage that requires cholesterol to begin with. Imagine that you have a cut on your arm and you put a bandage on it. Trying to manage cholesterol levels by simply reducing cholesterol in the blood is akin to ripping the bandage off rather than understanding what caused the cut and how we can make sure you don't get cut again. In their book, *Eat Fat, Lose Fat*, Mary Enig and Sally Fallon quote Dr. Meyer Texon pointing out that "indicting fat and cholesterol for hardening the arteries is like accusing white blood cells of causing infection, rather than helping the immune system to address it" (2006, 22).

Does diet affect cholesterol levels? Absolutely. Anything in your diet that causes damage or inflammation is going to have an effect on your cholesterol levels. But is it the dietary intake of cholesterol itself that affects those levels? In other words, is it the cholesterol in the yolk of the egg I had for breakfast that's responsible for higher cholesterol levels? Only somewhat, and not significantly. It is much more likely that it's the dietary intake of foods that cause inflammation and arterial damage—highly refined foods, excessive amounts of sugar, and overprocessed and rancid vegetable oils—that cause the damage, requiring your body to mobilize more cholesterol.

What this means is that a conversation about cholesterol is really a conversation about inflammation. Which bring me to the very important topic of essential fatty acids.

Essential Fatty Acids and Inflammation

We hear the term "essential fatty acids" tossed around, but what exactly does it mean? An essential fatty acid (EFA) is a fatty acid that your body cannot create from other fatty acids and thus is only accessible through diet. There are two types of EFA, both of which are polyunsaturated: alpha-linolenic (omega-3) and linoleic acid (omega-6).

Fatty acids, in particular EFAs, are intimately related to managing inflammation in the body. Fatty acids provide the building blocks for your body to make *prostaglandins*, agents that increase and decrease inflammation in the body. In a nutshell, saturated fats create the prostaglandins that increase inflammation and omega-6 and omega-3 create the prostaglandins that decrease inflammation. Both inflammation and anti-inflammation are important functions in our bodies, because they are the agents of healing. But as important as it is to be able to inflame (bring healing agents to a site of damage in your body), it is just as important to then be able to anti-inflame, removing those healing agents when they've done their job. We need to have a balance of both.

Both omega-3 and omega-6 are responsible for creating the prostaglandins that downregulate inflammation. *But*, the omega-6s we are eating are mostly highly industrialized and overprocessed oils such as corn, soybean, sunflower, safflower, and cottonseed. (Who decided eating a cotton by-product was a good idea?) "Highly industrialized" means damaged, which means it is inflammatory to the body, not anti-inflammatory. These are not the omega-6 oils that produce prostaglandins directly, such as borage, evening primrose, and black currant seed. The omega-6 oils we're eating are linoleic acid (LA), which needs to be conjugated into gamma-linolenic acid (GLA) in order to create the prostaglandins. This is a process that requires many cofactors, including the presence of magnesium and zinc, two very common nutritional deficiencies. The process is also inhibited by excess insulin and the consumption of trans-fatty acids, aspirin, alcohol, and NSAIDS (like ibuprofen), all extremely common. Furthermore, the ratio of omega-3 to omega-6 in our diet is skewed. Historically, the ratio was one to one. In the standard American diet, the ratio is now anywhere from one to fifteen to one to thirty.

A NOTE ABOUT OLIVE OIL AND INFLAMMATION

Olive oil, perhaps the most widely used and favored of all the vegetable oils, also plays a role in countering inflammation, but not because of its omega fatty acids. It has only very small amounts of the omega-6 fatty acid LA, and the remainder of its composition is monounsaturated and saturated fats. The reason olive oil (in particular, extra-virgin olive oil, which is unrefined and naked) is touted for its anti-inflammation properties is because it's jam-packed with powerful antioxidants, which, as their name suggests, inhibit oxidation.

What this means is we have significantly increased our body's ability to inflame but decreased our body's ability to anti-inflame. This is a big deal because inflammation is a significant health challenge and associated with many of the most common and chronic diseases we're currently seeing: heart disease (inflammation of the arteries), cancer, obesity, diabetes, Alzheimer's, and any of the many conditions ending in "-itis" (arthritis, colitis, bronchitis, and so on).

To rectify this balance, we need to increase our consumption of high-quality omega-3s and reduce our consumption of omega-6s. We need to balance the rest of our diets (eat naked) to ensure that our insulin levels are appropriate, that we have sufficient nutritional cofactors, and that we reduce inhibiting factors so that omega-6s can become the anti-inflammatory prostaglandins we so badly need.

Here's a table that shows those foods high in quality omega-3s and those high in quality omega-6s.

Good Sources of Essential Fatty Acids	
Omega-3	Omega-6
Oily fishes such as salmon, sardines, and anchovies	Sesame oil
Flaxseed oil	Peanut oil
Walnuts	Borage oil
Hemp seeds and hemp seed oil	Black currant seed oil
Pumpkin seeds and pumpkin seed oil	Evening primrose oil
Grass-fed beef	

In Summary

Isn't it great news that fat isn't bad? Now that you understand the basic science and nutritional importance of fats in your diet, here are the key take-away messages for making sure you're getting a good balance of high-quality naked fats in your diet:

- Quality is paramount. Because toxins are stored in fat, if budgeting food dollars, spend extra on high-quality fats and animal protein rather than worrying about organic produce.

- Having a good mix of all three types of fatty acid (saturated, monounsaturated, and polyunsaturated) in your diet is critical to maintaining good health.

- Store less stable vegetable oils in the refrigerator in tightly sealed containers that don't allow light. Never store oils near the stove.

- Scrupulously avoid any kind of transfats: partially or fully hydrogenated oils of any kind. These are found in many processed and packaged food products, so avoiding them completely and eating naked is your best bet.

- When cooking, never let a fat or oil smoke. This means it has gone rancid.

- Increase your consumption of omega-3s as much as possible by increasing the use of foods high in this fatty acid and considering supplementation. Strive for a one-to-one ratio of omega-3 to omega-6 in your diet.

A Quick Reference Guide to Naked Fats

Type of fat	Characteristics	Examples	Uses
Saturated	Stable Solid at room temperature.	Coconut oil Animal fats from grass-fed animals	Cooking and baking
Monounsaturated	Less stable Solid in the fridge, liquid at room temperature	Olive Oil Almonds and almond oil Avocados and avocado oil Pecans Cashews Peanuts and peanut oil	Cooking at very low temperatures Cold in dressings or on steamed veggies
Polyunsaturated	Least stable Liquid at room temperature and in the fridge	Fish oils Seed oils	Store in the refrigerator Cold in dressings or on steamed veggies

9

naked grains, beans, nuts, and seeds

I wrote this chapter while staying in Switzerland with friends, waking up most mornings to the smell of fresh-baked bread. Is there anything more intoxicating than the smell of bread baking!

Naked Grains

Bread and grains have long been a staple of our diet, and their importance runs deep through our culture. Unfortunately, as a quick trip through the bread aisle at your local grocery store will show, picking a bread to eat is not a simple task. The variety is endless and utterly confusing. Somehow we've taken one of the simplest foods, traditionally made of four basic ingredients (flour, yeast, water, and salt), and turned it into a fortified and refined nutritional mystery. My preference is to take it back to the basics. Let's start at the beginning, with the grain.

Whole Grains vs. Refined Grains

Grains are made up of three parts: the bran, the germ, and the endosperm. The bran is the outer layer or "shell," and its role is to protect the grain. It contains fiber, B vitamins, and minerals. The germ is the grain's core, the seed that has the capability of sprouting into a new plant. It contains antioxidants, more B vitamins, vitamin E, the minerals zinc and magnesium, and some protein and fats. The endosperm is the starchy part of the grain, its energy source. This is where the carbohydrates and most of the protein in the grain reside.

A truly whole grain or food made from whole grain includes all three parts: bran, germ, and endosperm. Refined grains or foods made from them include only one of the parts, usually the starchy endosperm. Generally speaking, a "white" grain product has had the germ and the bran removed, along with most of the nutritional value. There are a few exceptions to this rule (some rice, such as Arborio, is naturally white) but it's a good guideline.

Removing the nutrients from the grain has implications. On the upside, it makes things like bread doughy and spongy—textures we like and have come to crave. On the downside, the nutritional value of the food is severely compromised, and these stripped grain products actually deplete our body's reserves of important vitamins and minerals. The body needs the B vitamins found in the bran and germ of wheat to digest and absorb the wheat. With these vitamins removed, we must supply them from our own reserves, depleting our nutritional stores. It's because of this that nutrition expert Sally Fallon describes calories from such refined foods as "negative" calories, rather than simply "empty" calories—their net impact is negative since they deplete the body of important vitamins and minerals (Fallon 2001).

This is a big deal when you consider how much of our diet is based on foods made from refined grains. Author Marion Nestle estimates that "foods made from white flour account for nearly one-fifth of the calories in American diets" (2006, 485). And here she's only writing about white *flour*, not all the other "white" and otherwise refined foods we're consuming.

While most often we use the starch in the grain, it's not the only part that's sold separately. We should also consider bran products and wheat germ as refined foods. They have better nutritional press than white flour, but they're not whole.

The moral of the story? Choose foods made from whole grains. Even better, consume the whole grain itself, rather than foods made from it.

Whole brown rice is a better choice than pasta, even if the pasta is made from a whole grain.

Phytic Acid and the Importance of Proper Preparation

The conversation about whole versus refined isn't a new one. We're all familiar with it and most of us know that whole grains are preferable. What isn't as well-known is that it's important to prepare grains properly in order to receive their full nutritional benefit.

All grains, as well as beans, nuts, and seeds, have something called *phytic acid* in them. Phytic acid plays an important role as a protective coating that prevents the grain from breaking down prematurely. Ultimately, the grain's biological purpose isn't to make us delicious bread, but to create another plant. It's biologically designed to hold together until surrounded by moist, rich soil. Phytic acid keeps the grain fresh until it's in this environment.

A NOTE ABOUT BREAKFAST CEREALS

Arguably, the most common food we eat for breakfast is boxed breakfast cereal of one form or another. With few exceptions, these breakfast cereals are made using a process called *extrusion*, in which a slurry of grains is put through a machine called an *extruder*, which uses high temperatures and pressure to turn this slurry into cereals of different shapes and sizes: the "O"s, flakes, shredded bits, puffs, and so on. While no published studies have been done on the impact of extruded cereals on human health, the high heat and pressure damages the fatty acids, vitamins, and minerals and denatures the proteins, making them toxic. Granola can be an exception if you find some that uses only rolled oats (which aren't extruded), nuts, and seeds. However, no commercial brand that I'm aware of properly prepares its oats to neutralize the phytic acid and enzyme inhibitors.

To my mind, it simply makes logical sense to avoid boxed cereals because they're a processed food. Rolled or stone-cut oats are an exception to this rule, as they aren't extruded. I have included two breakfast cereal recipes in chapter 13, one hot and one cold. These use oats and are prepared using techniques that reduce the phytic acid.

THE MYSTERIOUS LOW-CARB BREAD PRODUCT

With the recent hype around low-carb diets, food manufacturers have, in typical fashion, risen to the challenge. How on earth can one take a carbohydrate, such as bread or a tortilla, and turn it into a "low-carb" food? Well, it's a bit of a misnomer, really. These products aren't necessarily low carb, but high soy. Often, the "low-carb" pronouncements on such products mean that soy—higher in protein, lower in carbohydrates—has been added to beef up the protein content of the food.

My advice: steer clear. If you're going to eat bread, eat bread. But have a nice, fresh loaf that's made of whole grain, ideally sprouted wheat or traditionally prepared sourdough.

Nutritionally speaking, phytic acid is an *antinutrient*, something in our food that interferes with the absorption of other nutrients. In this case, those nutrients are important minerals—iron, calcium, magnesium, copper, and zinc. Phytic acid binds with these minerals, making them unavailable to us. It also inhibits the enzymes pepsin, amylase, and trypsin, all of which are needed for the proper digestion of both protein and carbohydrates. This means it's more challenging for our bodies to digest our dinner when phytic acid is present (Nagel 2010).

The good news is that the phytic acid can be neutralized significantly by simple preparation techniques such as soaking, sprouting, and fermenting. We'll look at these three methods in depth in chapter 14, "Better Than Naked." Interestingly, many traditional methods of preparing grain included some kind of soaking, sprouting, or fermenting. Bulgur is made in the Middle East from coarsely ground sprouted wheat; in Scotland, oatmeal is made by soaking the oats overnight; and Ethiopians make their delicious and fragrant injera bread by fermenting teff.

The Gluten Problem

We looked at the topic of gluten in chapter 2, but to review, gluten is the primary protein in wheat, rye, and barley. This seemingly harmless protein has become one of the top allergens, and many people are sensitive to gluten without realizing it. This wouldn't be problematic if gluten weren't so ubiquitous in processed foods.

When we're talking about grains, it's helpful to identify those grains that do and don't contain gluten, so I've created quick-reference tables for you. If you believe you are sensitive or allergic to gluten, I've included some resources on my website (www.eatnakednow.com) to help you out. All of the recipes in this book are gluten free. The exception is two breakfast recipes that use oats, which don't themselves contain gluten but are often processed in facilities where cross-contamination is an issue.

Grains That Contain Gluten	
Barley	Barley is best known as a malt base for beer or as an ingredient in soups and stews.
Bulgur	Bulgur is wheat that has been parboiled, dried, and ground.
Couscous	Couscous has a healthy feel to it, but really it's just a pasta product made from refined flour. Whole-grain couscous is a healthier option, but it's still refined.
Kamut	Kamut is a type of wheat. It's an ancient grain, which means that it's been used for long periods throughout history without very much modification. It has more protein and a higher mineral content than most modern strains of wheat.
Wheat	The most abundant grain in our diet.
Spelt	Spelt is another ancient relative of wheat.
Rye	Rye is closely related to wheat and barley and is used for breads, beer, and whiskey.
Oats*	Oats are a special case when it comes to gluten. They themselves don't contain gluten, but they are often processed in facilities that also process gluten-containing grains, so there is an issue of cross-contamination. Truly gluten-free oats will be advertised as such. If you're sensitive to gluten, oats are probably fine in moderation. But if you have a full-blown allergy or celiac disease, avoid them unless they are specifically labeled as gluten free.

Gluten-Free Grains	
Amaranth	Amaranth is an Aztec grain that's high in protein. It tastes a little like corn.
Buckwheat	Despite having "wheat" in its name, buckwheat is actually no relation to wheat. Roasted buckwheat is called kasha. It's often used for pancakes or in soba noodles. If you're gluten intolerant, then read your labels carefully because many things made with buckwheat also have wheat in them. Often, if it is truly gluten free, the package will say so.
Millet	Millet has a nice, nutty flavor and is commonly used in India. It is particularly high in B vitamins.
Oats*	See the list of grains that contain gluten.
Quinoa	A favorite of many health advocates, quinoa is considered a superfood for its nutritional density in comparison to some other, more commonly used grains. It is high in protein and minerals, and because it's gluten free, it is widely tolerated. It comes most commonly in red and white, and more rarely in black. I like to make dishes using a combination of both.
Rice	Probably the most ubiquitous gluten-free grain, rice is easily digested, widely available, and comes in many interesting and flavorful varieties.
Teff	Teff, a staple in the northeastern African countries Ethiopia and Eritrea, is a type of millet. If you've eaten at an Ethiopian restaurant, you likely ate injera, a big pancakelike bread that's made from fermented teff.

Naked Beans

Ah, at last we come to a straightforward topic: beans. There's not a lot that's controversial or complicated about beans, and I like that. They're a good (if incomplete) source of vegetarian protein and can add a lot of variety and bulk to your meal at little additional cost. Perhaps their only potential offense is whether we've prepared them properly or not in order to make them more digestible. And when we haven't, the results are certainly entertaining, if a little uncomfortable.

There are many different and wonderful types of beans. Everything from red kidney, black, navy, garbanzo, pinto, adzuki, northeastern white… The list is long, varied, and delicious. I'm not going to go into the specific virtues and delights of each, but I encourage you to branch out and try some that are new to you.

When it comes to beans, it's all about proper preparation and the choice between canned or dried. The choice of canned or dried dictates the preparation, so let's start there.

Beans: Canned or Dried?

The choice between canned beans versus dried beans is really about how much time you've got before eating them. If it's 4 PM and you want beans in your dinner, then canned it is. There's simply no time to soak and cook dried beans properly in that time. If it's 4 PM and you want beans sometime tomorrow or this week, then you're set. Dried it is.

Nutritionally speaking, it's preferable to buy dried beans to soak and cook yourself. It doesn't actually take much of your time, just forethought and planning. With canned beans, you don't have control over how long or at what temperatures they've been cooked or how much salt was used in the preparation (and often, it's a lot). They will probably be digestible, but they may have been overcooked and overprocessed and thus have lost some of their nutritional value. If you're in a pinch, then canned is fine. It's one place I'm not that picky. If you are going to use canned beans, find the lowest-sodium variety you can.

EAT NAKED ON A BUDGET: CHOOSE DRIED BEANS

Dried beans are much cheaper than canned beans, becoming a truly affordable source of vegetarian protein. With a little planning, the process of soaking and cooking them can be easily integrated into your weekly meal preparation.

Proper Preparation of Beans

Beans, like the grains we just talked about, have phytic acid along with other powerful enzyme inhibitors in their skins. These prevent the absorption of minerals and make digestion of beans very difficult. It's these enzyme inhibitors and some hard-to-digest sugars that are responsible for the gas beans are notorious for creating. The solution is long periods of soaking and thorough cooking.

While most cooking instructions will say six to eight hours or overnight soaking is enough, it's actually quite helpful to soak beans for two to three days. Simply place the dried beans in a bowl with enough water to cover them by about four inches. Drain the water and replace it twice daily. When it's time to cook the beans, drain the water completely and add fresh water for cooking. You might find that a small tail has begun to form on some beans. This means that they have started sprouting and are even more digestible. We'll talk about the benefits of sprouting in chapter 14, "Better Than Naked."

Different beans have different cooking times, roughly dependent on their size. As a starting point, small beans such as lentils need, at minimum, thirty minutes; medium-sized beans such as adzuki and mung need at least sixty minutes; and large beans such as kidney and cannellini need a full hour and a half. Garbanzo beans (chickpeas) can require up to two and a half hours of cooking. Ultimately, you'll want to test the beans

A NOTE ABOUT SOY

We talked about soy at length in chapter 2. Soy has become the darling of many health-food advocates as a fairly complete, low-fat, and affordable source of vegetarian protein. Soybeans are used in an amazing array of foods, from the whole-bean edamame to classic tofu, soy milks, cheeses, and other faux animal foods like tofu dogs to widespread use in processed foods of all sorts.

Soy is the most difficult to digest of all the beans, bar none. In fact, the only way we can truly digest it is when it's fermented. Even soaking and sprouting aren't enough to break down its potent antinutrients. I recommend only consuming soy foods made from fermented soybeans. These include tempeh, miso, the traditional Japanese dish natto, and tamari or shoyu soy sauce. Steer clear of anything else. See chapter 2 for a more in-depth look at the ubiquitous soybean.

to make sure they're nice and soft. This is one instance in which overcooking is preferably to undercooking.

While these cooking times might sound really long, the nice thing about it is that beans don't require babysitting. You can put a pot of beans on the stove, bring it to a boil, and then turn down the heat to very low and leave it. I'd recommend staying in the house, but you don't have to be actively involved in the cooking.

Naked Nuts and Seeds

Nuts and seeds, much like beans, are a fairly uncomplicated and straightforward topic. They provide a delicious and interesting source of important fats in our diet and can be used in many creative ways. They're certainly one of my snacks of choice, and I use them liberally in salads and desserts.

Soaked, Roasted, or Raw?

As with grains and beans, nuts and seeds also contain antinutrients. In some cases, for example with flaxseeds, the levels of these antinutrients are so low that you really don't need to worry about it or do anything special. In these cases, eating the seed or nut raw is fine. In other cases, with the larger nuts such as cashews and almonds, for example, these antinutrients really should be neutralized before consuming them.

One way of neutralizing them is to slow roast the nuts. You can do this on a baking sheet in your oven at 200 degrees or by putting them dry (without oil or water) in a frying pan on low heat, shaking the pan often so that they don't burn. This certainly enhances their flavor significantly and has the handy nutritional benefit of neutralizing that phytic acid. This is the speediest way to deal with the antinutrients, but you're also reducing the nutritional value of the nut, damaging delicate enzymes and potentially damaging those unstable fatty acids.

There is a slightly more time-consuming approach that requires a little forethought and advanced planning. First, soak your nuts or seeds in filtered water overnight. Then, dry them on a baking sheet at the lowest temperature in your oven, ideally under 125 degrees. Even better, use a dehydrator to do this, as most ovens don't go below 170 degrees. This method has the benefit of neutralizing the enzyme inhibitors and actually

---

STORE NUTS AND SEEDS IN THE FRIDGE

Many people don't realize that nuts and seeds go rancid quickly. That jar of peanuts that's been sitting half full on your shelf for the last three years? Throw it out. If you remember from our discussion in chapter 8, "Naked Fats," nuts and seeds are high in those important but very delicate and unstable polyunsaturated fatty acids. The easy solution for this is to store nuts and seeds in the fridge.

---

waking up the enzymes themselves, making the nuts or seeds "living" foods and much more easily digested and used by our bodies. You can also soak the nuts overnight and then drain and rinse them, eating them without drying (expect the nuts to be softer than what you're used to). Stored in the refrigerator, these last up to a week. I like my almonds this way, but some folks find the taste of soaked almonds a little weird and prefer to have them dried.

So, the verdict on soaked, roasted, or raw? Well, the most important thing is that you buy the nuts raw and then do whatever you're going to do to them yourself. In other words, don't buy roasted nuts and assume the food company has done it for you. Avoid those nuts or seeds that come already roasted or flavored. It's highly likely that these have been heated to temperatures too high for the nuts and that the oils in them are rancid and the enzymes destroyed. At least when roasting at home you are in control of the variables. The best option is to soak the nuts and then dry them at very low temperatures. The next best is to lightly roast them yourself. If none of these techniques is possible, then eat them raw.

WHEN ORGANIC IS BEST

If it's possible, I recommend choosing organic nuts and seeds for the same reasons we discussed in chapter 4. That said, the only nuts I'd be adamant about buying organic are peanuts, as these are one of the most heavily sprayed crops. If you're able to find and afford all organic, that's fabulous. If not, prioritize peanuts and those nuts and seeds you eat most frequently.

In Summary

The key message about grains, beans, nuts, and seeds is essentially about proper preparation, a topic that's not often addressed in conversations about nutrition. If this feels really new and overwhelming to you, there are some easy places to start. For one, choose whole grains over processed products for your meals. For example, have whole, brown rice rather than pasta with your dinner, or try quinoa rather than couscous.

If that's something you already do, then try soaking a grain, bean, nut, or seed that you commonly use. I've included more information on how to do this in chapter 14. The most important thing with these foods is to start weeding out the foods in the "steer clear" row below, and start choosing the options in the "best" and "next best" rows.

Grains, Beans, and Nuts: Good, Better, Best			
	Grains	Beans	Nuts and Seeds
Best	Whole, sprouted	Soaked and cooked Fermented soy	Soaked and dried
Next best	Whole	Canned, low sodium	Home roasted
Okay		Canned	Raw
Steer clear	Cereals "Low-carb" bread products	Unfermented soy	Already roasted or seasoned

10
naked beverages, sweeteners, and condiments

When I think of beverages, sweeteners, and condiments, my mind immediately goes to soda pop, sweets, and ketchup. Of course, none of these typically qualify as naked, and, sure enough, a lot of beverages, sweeteners, and condiments are particularly "overdressed." The good news is that there are healthy, yummy, and easy alternatives that are naked. Yes, there's even such a thing as naked ketchup. But let's start first with drinks.

Naked Beverages

What we drink is an important part of our diet, and something we often don't give a lot of thought to. Did you know that the human body is approximately 70 percent water? We are mostly liquid, and so it's no surprise that the quality of the liquids we ingest has a big impact on our systems.

Wonderful Water

Would you be surprised if I told you that the biggest nutritional deficiency in North America is water? We are a culture of the chronically dehydrated. In his book *Your Body's Many Cries for Water* (1997), Dr. F. Batmanghelidj shows how so many of our chronic health complaints, from minor headaches to serious arthritis, can be linked back to dehydration.

Water is one of the most undervalued and important nutrients in our body. We are mostly water, and water is fundamental to every system and function in the body. We can survive without food for up to several weeks, but we can only survive without water for several days.

In my mind, water is the ideal naked beverage. It's abundant, it's (usually) free, it's easy, and it's really good for you. You can add things to it to change its flavor (see the Infused Water recipe in chapter 13, "Cook Naked" for some ideas here). It's truly refreshing, and it's a great pick-me-up. Try a glass of water instead of a cup of coffee next time you're having an energy dip in the afternoon—you might find you were just dehydrated, not actually in need of caffeine.

How Much Water?

Most of us don't drink enough water. But how much is enough? Well, that depends. The "eight glasses a day" standard advice is a little inaccurate because it doesn't account for our different sizes, different activity levels, and what else we're drinking. Dr. Batmanghelidj has created a simple formula to determine just how much water you should be drinking given certain factors. Take your body weight in pounds and divide that number in half. That's the total number of ounces of water you need to drink on a daily basis *before* any diuretic beverages or strenuous exercise. For example, if you weigh 120 pounds, you need to drink 60 ounces of water a day. If you drink a diuretic beverage (coffee, tea, pop, juice, a sugary drink, or alcohol), you need to drink the equivalent of one and a half to two times the volume of the diuretic beverage just to offset its effects. So, if you drink an 8-ounce cup of coffee, you'll need to drink at least 12 to 16 ounces of water to make up for it—and that's on top of the 60 ounces (or whatever your specific amount is) of water you're drinking as a daily minimum. The maximum water you should drink in a day is a gallon (128 ounces), so if you're quite heavyset and drink a lot of diuretic beverages, you might have to tweak this formula a little.

A NOTE ABOUT FILTERS

The topic of water filters could fill up its own chapter, as there are so many different options and varieties. There's everything from your basic Brita filter to the complex multi-thousand-dollar filtration systems that balance the pH and exact mineral content. This is clearly more than we have room for here.

My advice is that decent water is better than no water, and filtering your own is ultimately more affordable than buying bottled (let alone the environmental cost of all that plastic). I use a basic home system that filters all the bad stuff out and then rests the water on mineral stones to put the good stuff—the minerals your body needs to use the water—back in. It was affordable and has lasted for years.

The only water I will advise you to use with caution is reverse-osmosis and distilled water. Both of these are extremely pure, and while absent of all possible contaminants, they're also devoid of the minerals needed for your body to actually use the water. If you drink reverse-osmosis or distilled water, be sure to add minerals back in so that you don't unintentionally leach them from your body's stores.

You're Not Hungry, You're Thirsty

One of the things that happens when we're chronically dehydrated is that we don't actually realize we're thirsty. We often mistake our body's thirst for hunger and eat when we just need to drink some water. If you find yourself reaching for a snack between meals, drink a glass of water first. Let it sit for about ten minutes and see if you're still hungry. If you are, grab that snack. If you're not, then you weren't really hungry after all, just thirsty.

Pop Goes the World

Pop is one of the topics in nutrition that can really get a rise out of me. There's nothing redeeming about it. It's loaded with sugar—or worse, artificial sweeteners—it's nutritionally void, and it messes with your body's balance of minerals. It's something we reach for when we're thirsty, but not only does it *not* satisfy that thirst, it dehydrates us further because it's a diuretic. Soda is often packed full of caffeine and a whole slurry of artificial flavors and flavor enhancers. And it can be really, really addictive. I have spent months working with clients to ease them out of a Diet Coke habit, and it's a long, painful process.

Basically, I steer clear of the stuff and I highly encourage you to do the same. If you like a fizzy flavored beverage, especially on a hot day, try drinking Sparkling Flavored Soda from the recipe in chapter 13. It's just as refreshing as any pop out there without the downsides of pop. Another great and healthy option is kombucha, a traditional fermented green tea that's slightly fizzy from the fermentation process. Kombucha has gained popularity in recent years, and it's usually available in health-food stores.

Coffee and Teas

One of the questions I get asked a lot is about coffee. Health friend or foe? Well, it depends, and, as with so many things in the field of nutrition, there is a lot of disagreement on the topic.

First of all, it depends on what coffee you're drinking. A small cup of organic, shade-grown coffee with a dash of real cream isn't going to be the end of the world. An extra-large mocha latte with lots of sugar, artificial flavors, and extra whipped cream—well, that's a different story. If you love your coffee and don't want to give it up, limit it to one small cup in the morning, and keep it simple. Drink it black or with a little real cream (none of that fat-free creamer that has lots of chemicals and artificial flavors to make you think you're drinking something yummy).

Of course, it's even better to simply avoid coffee altogether. With its high levels of caffeine, drinking it is our body's equivalent to running on fumes. Jacked up on caffeine, you end up depleting your true energy stores and, over time, are at risk of exhaustion. Coffee might provide a quick boost in the short term, but it's draining in the long run. It's also damaging to the lining of the intestine, responsible for the "elimination response" for which it is renowned.

What About Decaffeinated?

Generally, I don't recommend decaffeinated coffee. This is because the process used to remove the caffeine is arguably more toxic than the caffeine itself and can leave up to 60 percent of the caffeine in the beans. The best option for decaffeinated coffee is the Swiss Water Process. It's a

ORGANIC AND FAIR TRADE

With coffee in particular, choosing organic is important. Coffee is one of the most heavily sprayed crops, so choosing organic makes a significant difference. If you want to feel even better about your purchase, choose organic *and* certified fair-trade coffee. The Fair Trade Certified label "guarantees consumers that strict economic, social, and environmental criteria were met in the production and trade of an agricultural product," as explained on the TransFair USA website (www.transfairusa.org/content/certification).

much gentler and more natural process using only water and removes 99.9 percent of the caffeine.

And What About Tea?

Tea is a great alternative to coffee, in particular the antioxidant-rich green and white teas. These have lower levels of caffeine, so they're gentler on your system. And because tea is made by steeping leaves in water, it doesn't have the potentially negative health effects associated with the roasting process that's involved with coffee. Even better are herbal teas, which typically have soothing, mild flavors and no caffeine.

Now, as with coffee, how naked your tea is depends on how you're drinking it. Plain is best, and adding a little naked milk is next best. I would avoid loading it up with lots of sugar and other stuff. A recent phenomenon is tea lattes made using prebrewed and already sweetened teas. These are just as packed with sugar and artificial flavors as you'll find in the un-naked coffees. Also, be wary of bottled iced teas that have added flavors and sweeteners. Enjoy a homemade version instead. See the recipe for Iced Green Tea in chapter 13.

Juice

Juice is one of those beverages that sounds so innocent and nutritious. Take some fruit and squeeze out the good stuff. Images of a bright sunny morning and a cold glass of orange juice sparkling on the table run through my mind. What could be harmful in that? Well, juice, especially fruit juice, is actually not as healthy as you might think.

First of all, juice is mostly sugar. Yes, it's sugar that comes from fruit, but as soon as you juice the fruit you're removing all the fiber that comes with that sugar and slows down its absorption. You're also consuming far more sugar than you would if you were to simply eat the whole fruit. It takes up to eight oranges to make one glass of orange juice. That's a lot of oranges. My guess is that you wouldn't normally sit down and eat eight oranges. Maybe two, if they're particularly yummy and you're particularly hungry. But more than that is usually too much. When you're drinking a glass of orange juice, you're getting the sugar of all of those oranges without the fiber that comes with it.

Commercially made juice is also pasteurized, just like dairy. The heat kills off any potential pathogens, and unfortunately also damages the more delicate nutrients in the fruit. This means you're getting all the sugar without the fiber and without the full nutritional value of the fruit. And sometimes, amazingly, juice makers add more sugar. So really, drinking juice is only slightly more healthy than drinking pop. I avoid it completely.

What about freshly juiced juice? Well, this is the only time I'd recommend drinking juice, if you must drink it. Juice the fruit yourself, drink it immediately, and drink it sparingly. The nutritional value of juice deteriorates really rapidly, so the sooner you drink it, the better. The same goes for vegetable juices. Ideally, you'd eat the whole vegetable. But if you really like the juice, then invest in your own juicer and drink what you've juiced as soon as it's made.

Naked Sweeteners

Sugar has been a big target of health practitioners in recent years, and for good reason. The list of arguments for avoiding it is long, and the list of harmful effects in your body even longer. Part of the problem with sugar is that we're eating so much of it. In 1700, when sugar was a rarity and only for the wealthy, average consumption was at approximately 4 pounds per year. By 1900 that number had risen to 90 pounds per year, and in 2008, more than half of Americans consumed a half pound of sugar *daily*. That's 180 pounds of sugar per year (Johnson and Gower 2008). These outrageous levels of sugar consumption are an enormous part of the health problem in North America today, quite directly responsible for obesity, diabetes, and a host of degenerative diseases. To understand why sugar is so hard on the body, let me take a moment to explain how your body manages energy levels and what consuming all this sugar is doing to you.

The Impact of Sugar

The human body has a very small allowable range when it comes to the amount of sugar in the blood. Anything nearing the upper limits triggers the secretion of *insulin*, the hormone that tells your body to store the excess sugar as glycogen for later use. Anything nearing the lower limit triggers the secretion of *glucagon*, the hormone that tells your body to release some of the glycogen you've stored. In an ideal scenario—one in which you're eating balanced meals with lots of vegetables, some good-quality protein, and some good, healthy fats, with very little, if any, sugar—the ebb and flow of your body managing these blood sugar levels is barely noticeable. You feel great after meals, your energy levels are nice and even, and as a really nice side benefit, your waistline is trim. Unfortunately, the ideal scenario is a rarity.

What's much more common, to the point of becoming "normal," is that we consume way too much sugar, starting right from the get-go. A fairly typical North American breakfast is a glass of juice (sugar), a bagel with some peanut butter and jam (the bagel is essentially sugar, with a little fat and protein topped with more sugar), and maybe a coffee to go with it (caffeine, maybe with a little fat and often with more sugar). Swap out the bagel with a bowl of cereal and you have basically the same breakfast.

When you start your day off this way your blood sugar levels go screaming up out of range (what a rush!), and your body needs to go into overdrive to get those levels back within range again. Pump-pump-pump goes your pancreas, secreting loads of insulin to pull out all that excess sugar to be stored for later use (some of which is stored as glycogen and the rest as fat). The problem is that the insulin is so good at its job, the next thing you know you're hurtling down into a sugar crash, far past the bottom limits of your blood sugar range. Most unfortunately, the glycogen stores can't be released fast enough to bring your blood sugar levels back up before you're launched into another state of emergency. This time, your body tries to rescue the situation by releasing the stress hormones cortisol and adrenaline. Often, even these hormones aren't enough to do the trick, and thus you get that strong craving for more sugar or a strong cup of coffee. And the cycle repeats.

This is such a normal way of being that we've got whole social structures organized around it. Enter the midmorning and midafternoon coffee break. When you're not eating sugar, you don't need the coffee break—or at least you don't need the coffee and sweet treat. You could do with some water or a cup of tea and maybe a handful of nuts.

The side effects of this dizzying cycle aren't to be ignored. It's a major factor in weight gain, elevated triglycerides, increased LDL and VLDL (the more harmful types of cholesterol), and lowered HDL, the "good" cholesterol (Reiser 1985; Liu et al. 2000). It leads to hypoglycemia (Kelsay et al. 1974; Thomas et al. 1982), metabolic syndrome, and ultimately, diabetes (Beck-Nielsen, Pedersen, Schwartz-Sørensen 1978; Reiser et al. 1986). It speeds up aging (Van Boekel 1991). It creates its own vicious cycle of sugar cravings (Colantuoni et al. 2002), negatively affecting your mood and sometimes leading to depression (Christensen 1991). It suppresses your immune system (Sanchez 1973), it has been linked to several types of cancer (Moerman, Bueno de Mesquita, and Runia 1993; De Stefani et al. 1998; Cornée et al. 1995), and it can cause headaches (Grant 1979)... I could go on, but do I need to?

It is for all these reasons that sugar is essentially *not* a naked food. As much as you can, steer clear. I was raised in a family where dessert was a nightly affair. I developed quite the sweet tooth over the years, to the point where I would go out of my mind if I couldn't have my midafternoon chocolate fix. A bowl of candy next to me didn't last longer than a few minutes, regardless of its size. I always saved room for dessert, and if I didn't, I stuffed it into an overfull belly anyway, only regretting that I'd eaten so much of my main course. I was wildly hypoglycemic and would fall dramatically into what I called my "sugar coma" multiple times a day, which was then cause for consuming more sugar.

Life after sugar looks very different. Amazingly to me, desserts don't really appeal. I'll treat myself once in a while, but often a couple of bites will do me just fine. More often than not, I'll pass. Things that didn't taste sweet before, like certain vegetables, are now just scrumptious. My energy levels are nice and consistent throughout the day (no more crazy spikes and crashes), and I don't feel the need for a nap after my meals anymore. And did I mention that I'm often in a much better mood as a result?

Dessert Options

The best solution when it comes to sugar is to eliminate it, if not completely, as much as possible. My vote is to bring sugar and desserts back to their role as treats for special occasions, not a daily habit or, dare I say, an addiction. When there is occasion (hopefully rare) for something a little sweet, here are some sweeteners that I prefer and would call naked. As a general rule, choose those that are as unrefined as possible. This will mean that they have some nutritional value in addition to a sweet taste. Also, some sugars have a lower glycemic load than others, which means they convert to glucose in the blood at a slower rate. Here are some options to choose from:

- **Raw honey.** Only for use cold (don't cook or bake with it), raw honey is a natural antibacterial, antiviral, and antifungal. It's worth the extra effort to find raw honey, as pasteurization damages its delicate nutrients and beneficial enzymes.

- **Unsulphured, blackstrap molasses.** This liquid by-product of the process of refining sugar is sweet while also high in minerals.

- **Rapadura.** This is dried juice of the sugarcane, and as unrefined as you'll get when it comes to sugar.

- **Maple syrup.** Splurge and get the real stuff. I like the lower grades, because the maple flavor is stronger. It's rich in minerals, and being Canadian, I'll admit I have a bias for this one.

- **Stevia.** This sweet herb makes a nice and soothing tea if you use the whole leaf, and the powder made from it has become a favorite of many health practitioners because it has negligible impacts on blood sugar and zero calories. Use sparingly—a little goes a long way.

- **Coconut sugar.** This sugar is made from coconut blossoms, has a low glycemic load, and is only minimally refined. It's high in minerals and B vitamins, and works well in baking.

- **Dates.** Dates are nice and sweet and packed with minerals. If you need to sweeten a sauce or a dressing, throw a pitted date into your food processor or blender, and it'll do the trick. Talk about unrefined!

Naked Condiments

Ah, condiments. Where to begin? So many kinds, so many brands, so many labels to read. And, unfortunately, that's often what it comes down to on this topic. Condiments are where a lot of processed items sneak into our diets. I've watched absolutely delicious and nutritious salads be drowned in store-bought salad dressing filled with low-quality oils, sugar, and loads of artificial flavors. I've seen otherwise nutrient-packed omelets get smothered in ketchup, or veggie sticks get dipped into a pot of dip that was really just hydrogenated oils and lots of additives. And it made my heart sink a little.

From the ketchups and mayos to the mustards and salad dressings, your absolute best bet is to make it yourself. Yes, ketchup can be homemade and even quite nutritious! It was once a health-promoting food made using fermentation techniques rather than just lots of sugar (Fallon 2001). I've included several basic condiment recipes in chapter 13, such as hummus, pesto, and a couple of simple and tasty salad dressings. Check them out. They're easier than you might think. And when you make it yourself, you have total control over ingredients and quantities.

What to do if you can't make a condiment yourself for lack of time and planning? Well, this is where you become a label reader and avoid the worst offenders. Steer clear of anything that has high-fructose corn syrup, any kind of partially or fully hydrogenated oil, artificial sweeteners, and soy (unless it's tamari soy sauce or miso, both of which are fermented). If you can easily pronounce and recognize the ingredients on the label, that's a good thing. If sugar in any of its forms appears in the first five ingredients, it's probably best to put the condiment back on the shelf.

To make the transition to naked condiments, here's what I'd suggest you do. Pick the condiment you use most often at your home and learn how to make it yourself. You don't have to throw out everything in your refrigerator door right away. Just pick the one you use most often and start there. Once you've learned how to make it yourself, you can move on to another one. Over time, you'll realize that there's no need to trek down that aisle in the grocery store, and your food will taste much fresher and healthier in the process.

In Summary

While some un-naked ingredients can sneak their way into our drinks, sweet treats, and condiments, there are certainly naked versions of all of these that are just as tasty and much better for our health. In terms of beverages, start by drinking more water and eliminating or greatly reducing anything in the "steer clear" section in the table on the next page. For your sweeteners, replace refined sugar and artificial sweeteners with the natural sweeteners I mentioned above. Experiment to find the ones you like best. For your condiments, slowly transition over to making your own, and when you buy them ready-made, look for those with the fewest and nakedest ingredients.

Beverages, Sweeteners, and Condiments: Good, Better, Best

	Beverages	Sweeteners	Condiments
Best	Water Herbal or green teas Naturally fermented beverages like kombucha	Raw honey Unsulphured, blackstrap molasses Rapadura Maple syrup (not Grade A) Stevia Coconut sugar Dates	Homemade from naked ingredients
Next best	Sparkling mineral water Black tea Freshly juiced vegetable juice	Pasteurized honey Grade A maple syrup	Store-bought, with only naked ingredients on the label
Okay	Coffee (preferably organic, shade-grown; if decaf, then Swiss Water Process) Unpasteurized, fresh-squeezed fruit juice, in small amounts only	Agave (low glycemic but highly refined and high fructose content)	
Steer clear	Soda pop of any type (diet or regular) Pasteurized juice	Refined sugar (includes "brown" sugar, which is still refined) Artificial sweeteners	Any condiments with high-fructose corn syrup, hydrogenated oils, soy, or ingredients you can't pronounce

PART 2

how to get naked

11

transitioning to a naked diet

By this point you've got a pretty good sense of what I'm talking about when I say "eat naked." You might be looking at your own diet and realizing that it's a little "overdressed." Don't panic. No matter how great the distance might seem between how you're eating now and eating naked, the gap is certainly one you can close.

Change is never instantaneous—it's a process that builds over time. This might not be what you want to hear. I know it's something I struggle with. "But I want to be there *now!*" is my first instinct when learning new information and seeing the possibilities for a new way of being.

True and lasting change takes time. It just does. Kind of like building new muscles, change of any kind is a process of creating new habits to replace old ones. We need to embrace and accept the fact that it's a gradual endeavor and simply take that first step. As you begin to shift your diet to eating naked, I really encourage you to be easy with it. Go at your own pace, be gentle on yourself, and relax in the knowledge that you have plenty of time to change.

One Meal at a Time

The real key to transitioning from your current diet to eating naked is to pick one place at a time to make adjustments. This can be one meal, be it breakfast, lunch, dinner, or snacks, or it can be one type of ingredient, such as veggies, fats, or meats.

Let's say you decide to start with breakfast. Personally, this is my favorite place to start because how you begin the day affects everything that comes after it. What's your typical breakfast? Maybe it's a bowl of cereal with milk. Maybe it's a bagel with cream cheese, a glass of orange juice, and a cup of coffee. Maybe it's a breakfast bar that you grab as you rush out the door. Maybe you like the greasy-spoon-style bacon and eggs.

Whatever your breakfast is, consider how you could make it more naked. If you eat cereal for breakfast, now you know about proper grain preparation. If you start your day with a bowl of cereal, try some homemade muesli rather than what comes out of the box. If you eat instant oatmeal, try making your own, having soaked the oats the night before. If you like eggs and bacon for breakfast, look at the quality of the eggs you're eating and consider replacing the bacon with some veggies.

If you don't want to start with a whole meal, start with something you eat often. For example, let's say you're a salad lover who buys dressing from the store. A good place to add more naked to your diet would be to start making your own dressing. That's one simple change you can make that will have a big impact.

You can also do a scan of your eating habits, looking for the worst offenders. What in your diet offers the least nutritional value and is something you eat often? Is it potato chips to get you through the afternoon? Do you drink lots of diet soda? Choose something you reach for often but that probably isn't the healthiest thing you could eat. How can you replace that with something more naked?

Try One Recipe from This Book a Week

If you're not interested in sleuthing through your current diet to find things you can tweak, here's an easy way to slowly transition to eating naked. Try one new recipe from this book each week, and then make it for two or three weeks. If you're able to do this consistently every week, you'll have over forty new meals under your belt and a whole new way of cooking integrated into your life. This is a great complement to the one-meal-at-a-time strategy, especially if you're not sure where to begin.

Make It Your Own

Once you've tried a new recipe, make it again a couple of times. Once you've figured it out and it feels natural, try changing it up a bit. Maybe you've made the enchiladas from this book, and instead of black beans you want to try pinto beans. Go for it! Maybe you want to add a favorite vegetable. Maybe you want to add some ground beef (grass fed, of course). Make it your own. Once you've been using the recipe for a while, you might be inspired to change it, add to it, or take something out. That's when things get exciting.

How Naked Is Your Dinner?

Run your dinner through the naked test. Is it made from fresh ingredients? Are they organic? Are the veggies local? Is the meat from pastured animals or industrial? What kind of fats are you using? Slowly, one ingredient at a time, see how you can make your dinner more naked.

Making changes to meals you currently prepare is a great trick for family favorites. I have a client who had pizza with her family every Friday night. When we first started working together, they ordered in a couple of pizzas from the closest and cheapest chain. Not so naked. We shifted them first to eating a storebought pizza that they baked themselves, then to premade crust and naked toppings, assembled and baked at home. Before

---

HAVE A NAKED DINNER PARTY

Everything's more fun when you make it a party, right? Involve your friends and community and have a naked dinner party. Take some of the pressure off yourself and make it potluck. Let people know that the only requirements are that the ingredients for what they're bringing are fresh, in season, and whole, and that they make it themselves. You can add a twist and ask that they get at least half of the ingredients from a farmers' market. Make it fun and enjoy the experience together.

---

long, they had turned pizza night into a full-on pizza-making party where they used all fresh, local produce and meats for toppings, used homemade pesto for the pizza sauce, and even used crust they'd made themselves and saved in batches, stored in the freezer. The whole family got involved, and each person made his or her own custom pizza. Yes, it's a little more work than just ordering in, but so much healthier and so much more educational for the kids, and it added a whole new element to their family Friday nights.

Add More Veggies

As I mentioned earlier in the book, you really can't overdo it on veggies. I've never encountered a client who didn't need more veggies in his or her diet. Even the strict vegetarians were often, ironically, not eating enough veggies. If you're not interested in overhauling what you eat right now, then start by adding in more veggies.

Strive to fill at least half, if not 75 percent, of your plate with veggies. Have some raw, some cooked. If you add a salad to lunch and dinner, there's a good number of raw veggies right there. I like to have at least one thing that's green on my plate at every meal. One green veggie and one colorful is a really good start. Always make more veggies than you need. If you're going to go back for seconds, fill up on more veggies. With few exceptions, most of the recipes in this book have at least 50 percent veggies, so simply following these recipes will give you some ideas on how to boost your veggie intake.

Slow Down and Sit Down

What you're eating is only part of the story of eating naked. Surprised? Well, it's been shown that all sorts of factors influence how your body absorbs the food you're eating, and it's got as much to do with how you eat as what you eat. Interestingly, changing one often leads to changing the other.

Let me share some basic physiology, which was new to me when I started exploring the intricacies of digestion. Digestion is regulated by your *autonomic nervous system*, the subconscious nervous system that controls and regulates those functions in your body you don't have to think about, like your heart beating or your lungs breathing. You have some conscious control of these functions—for example, you can consciously change the depth of your breath. But if you stop thinking about it, you don't stop breathing. Digestion is the same way. You don't have to remember to break down the food once you've swallowed it—your body takes care of it.

There are two parts to your autonomic nervous system: the parasympathetic nervous system and sympathetic nervous system. The *parasympathetic nervous system* is your rest-and-relaxation response. The *sympathetic nervous system* is your fight-or-flight response, the stress response. When you're in a parasympathetic state, your body is relaxed and digestion flows smoothly. Your body can only heal when it's in the parasympathetic state. On the other hand, when your sympathetic nervous system is dominant, your body is on high alert. Energy and blood are diverted from "nonessential" functions, such as digestion and healing, to the urgent matter at hand. It's an important survival mechanism, designed to protect us when we're in danger.

What's interesting about this is how the body defines stress. As Marc David, nutritionist, psychologist, and author of *The Slow Down Diet* (2005), explains, stress is the body's response to any threat, whether that threat is real or perceived. I believe the important word here is "perceived." The body mounts the same physiological response whether we're annoyed sitting in traffic or running away from a woolly mammoth. It might not be quite to the same degree, but the response is the same. And this response shuts down your digestion.

This means that if you're eating while under stress, your body will have a really difficult time digesting and absorbing that food. How many of us are eating under stress? Most of us. And to make matters worse, stress causes spikes in cortisol and insulin, hormones that tell our bodies to store fat.

The best and easiest way to minimize stress, especially while we're eating, is to sit down to eat, eat slowly, and actually be present for the meal. This might seem overly simple, but don't underestimate the power of eating a meal in a relaxed, calm state of mind, really savoring every mouthful and thoroughly enjoying the experience. So, if you're struggling to change *what* you eat, then start by changing *how* you eat.

Do you eat quickly? Try eating slowly. Put your fork down between bites, and don't pick it up again until you have completely chewed and swallowed the first mouthful. Take big breaths between bites.

Do you eat standing up or rushing out the door on your way to work? Take ten minutes to sit down to eat. Those ten minutes could be the difference between your breakfast satisfying you or leaving you hungry again in a couple of hours.

Do you notice what you're eating, or is eating part of your multitasking? Try really paying attention to the tastes, the flavors, and the experience of eating your food.

We are biologically wired to seek pleasure and avoid pain, and feeding ourselves, a deeply nourishing and sensual act, can be a vital part of that pleasure-seeking experience. If your body is looking for pleasure all day long and you're either not giving it any or you're so busy you didn't notice it, then it's going to keep looking for that pleasure. The primary way your body satisfies the need for pleasure is to tell you it's still hungry (David 2005).

Kitchen Cleanout

I'm a big fan of not putting myself in front of temptation. If something is in the cupboards and I'm hungry, I'll probably eat it. To make sure I don't make decisions that I'll regret later, I don't have anything in my cupboards that I don't want to eat.

To get to this place, I've had to do several big kitchen-cupboard cleanouts. This involves me on a stool, taking everything out of the cupboards and fridge, and only putting back those things that are truly naked or that are rare, special treats (be very careful here).

Why is the cleanout so important? Well, here's the scenario. You've had a long day at work, your boss was in a mood and you were the target, and the kids are overtired and snarky. You get home and open the cupboards to make dinner. Let's say your comfort food of choice is potato chips. If you open the cupboards and there's a bag of chips staring you in the face, what's the chance, at that moment, of you simply reaching past them to get the other ingredients you need for dinner? It becomes a matter of willpower, and quite honestly, I think that's setting you up for failure. If you open the cupboard and there's no bag of potato chips, you're setting yourself up to simply make dinner, because there's no temptation staring you in the face in that moment.

A kitchen cleanout is a great exercise to do once or twice a year. Make it part of your spring cleaning. It feels good to do a big reorganization, clean, and purge of things that don't support your desires to be healthy, fit, and a size you feel proud of. I like to make an event of it. I'll turn on some music, make a big pitcher of iced tea, throw on an apron, and go for it.

In Summary

There are many different ways to move from your current diet to a naked one. Perhaps you prefer the more radical approach of a big kitchen clean-out, simply replacing any non-naked foods in your kitchen with naked ones. Or maybe you're so busy right now that you really can't fathom changing what you eat, so you start with eating a little more slowly and noticing your food more. It could be that you like to do things methodically, like me, and you've decided to pick one new recipe a week to help you slowly learn and build new habits in the kitchen.

How you do it is completely up to you. There's no one right approach. Each of us is different and makes change in our own way, at our own pace. The important thing is that you know where you're headed and that you take the next doable step. If you persist, before you know it you'll be eating naked, and overprocessed foods will be a thing of the past.

12
shop naked

It's sad but true that one of the hardest places to find real, whole food is at the supermarket. So much of what lines the aisles and stocks the shelves isn't really food, it's what Michael Pollan so eloquently and appropriately calls "edible foodlike substances" (2009, 1). If not at the supermarket, where to find naked food?

Clearly, an integral part of the whole eat-naked experience is actually finding and procuring naked food. Where you live will have a certain influence over the best places to find it readily and affordably, but there are some standard places to look.

Your Local Farmers' Market

A fantastic resource for truly naked food is your local farmers' market. Shopping here is the ultimate way to shop naked. Finding local and seasonal food is easy, and you get to buy it directly from the farmers themselves. What better way to spend a lazy summer weekend morning than perusing the stands at the farmers' market, tasting and trying new things and talking to the producers about the food? It's far more than just a boring old trip to the grocery store. You can make it an outing for the whole family. It's a weekend ritual at our home. Many farmers' markets have live music, all sorts of fun stuff like face painting and special treats for the kids, and, of course, an abundance of freshly picked local food. The sense of community is powerful. Little kids running around, folks out with their cloth grocery bags overstuffed with fresh produce, bumping into neighbors and gushing over a particularly scrumptious blackberry. Shopping isn't a chore here—it's an event.

One of my favorite things about the farmers' market is the connection it fosters between you and the farmer who grew your food. Buying something all sterilized and prepackaged at the store, where you have no idea who grew, picked, or prepared your food, keeps us far removed from the actual act of growing it. At the farmers' market, the person selling you the food is more often than not the one who grew it. This benefits you because you can ask the farmers about the farming practices they use. It's also great for the farmers, who get a close relationship with their customers and ultimately earn more because there's no middleman skimming off the top of their profits.

Farmers' markets are also a terrific way to expand your food horizons and entice you to try new things or new varieties of familiar things. Many stands will have samples that you can taste right on the spot. At one of the many markets here in Los Angeles, there's a stand that currently has samplings of five or six different kinds of pluot (a *pluot* is a hybrid of a plum and an apricot). You can taste each one and pick your perfect flavor. Fruity and sweet, or tangy and a little sour? You won't find that kind of variety at your typical grocer.

Community Supported Agriculture

Community supported agriculture (known as a CSA) is basically an arrangement that you have with a farmer where you share the risk and reward of the farming season. Typically it's set up where the farmer offers a set number of shares to people in the community at the beginning of the season. These shares cover the expenses of running the farm and growing the food. In return, you receive a box of the fresh harvest every week throughout the summer.

CSAs are excellent ways of connecting directly to farmers and ensuring your access to consistently local, seasonal, and ultrafresh food. You'll get exposure to fruits and vegetables that might be new to you and develop a close relationship with the farmer who's growing your food. The farmer gets the benefit of cash in at the beginning of the season when it's needed most and can focus on growing the food rather than finding a market for it during peak season. I've included some resources for how to find a CSA in your area on my website: www.eatnakednow.com.

Organic Grocery Delivery Services

Organic grocery delivery services are a relatively recent phenomenon. They're a great resource for people who are committed to eating naked but don't have the time to shop for the food *and* prepare it. These delivery services make grocery shopping a process that you can do online, and they bring your groceries right to your door. Increasingly, these services bring more to you than just organic produce—several now offer everything from toilet paper to grass-fed beef—and you have some flexibility of choice over what actually arrives in your box. Perhaps broccoli is in season but you've had enough broccoli for now. You have the option to forgo items, whereas with many CSAs, you have less control over what's coming to you. I've been using one of these services (Spud!) for years, and I'm a huge fan. It complements my trips to the farmers' market and makes sure I still eat really high-quality, local food when I don't have time for a run to the store.

Grocers with a Specific Commitment to Naked Foods

The tremendous success of a grocery chain such as Whole Foods is a testament to the increased demand for naked foods. Grocers such as this, with a specific and overt commitment to supplying high-quality, locally sourced, organic food, are becoming hugely popular and widely available. These stores are particularly responsive to customer requests, so if you're looking for something and can't find it, be sure to ask.

Something to remember when you're shopping at one of these grocers is that, even though they have made an express commitment to supplying healthier foods, just because they supply it doesn't mean it's naked. You still need to apply the principles of naked food—fresh, whole, unprocessed, unrefined, organic if possible, and ideally local. A common mistake is to assume that because a food is available at a health-food store that means it's a health food. This isn't always the case.

Conventional Supermarkets

Although they might not have the variety or the quantity, more conventional supermarkets are starting to stock naked foods. The organics section, formerly nonexistent or tucked away in a corner with rather soggy-looking lettuce and a couple of bags of apples, is now expanding, stocked with fresher produce and displayed more prominently. I recently saw grass-fed beef at a large chain store and have noticed raw-milk cheeses in some unlikely places.

My advice to you when shopping at a conventional supermarket is to stay as much as possible on the perimeter of the store. This is where the freshest, most naked food tends to be stocked, and you won't be tempted by all the novelties, fancy packaging, and wild nutritional promises that are found on the more processed foods. As a general rule, if a food is advertising all its health benefits, it's probably not that naked. A stalk of broccoli or a piece of raw-milk cheese speaks for itself and doesn't need all that advertising. Be wary of large claims and health promises. Often that means something was done to the food that made it require special advertising.

What About the Really Hard-to-Find Stuff?

Some naked foods, for example raw milk or eggs from pastured chickens, can be much harder to find than, say, organic carrots and broccoli. In the case of raw dairy products, this is largely due to strict legislation around pasteurization. In the case of things like eggs from pastured chickens or grass-fed beef, this is largely due to the still relatively small demand and supply. While it can be more of a challenge to find these foods, it's certainly not impossible. And in fact, if you have the interest and energy for it, I encourage you to take the time to sleuth it out. Voting with our dollars is a powerful way to signal food producers of our needs and wants, and it's deeply satisfying to find a new, great source of delicious, naked food.

In the case of raw milk, you might not be able to buy it at a grocery store, but you might be able to find a farmer from whom you can buy it directly. You may even be able to invest in what's called a "cow share," where you own a part of the cow and in return receive fresh milk from it weekly. The best resource for finding a source of raw dairy is www.real-milk.com. I've also listed some other resources on my website.

In the case of pastured chickens or grass-fed beef, you can often find these at organic grocers, food cooperatives, or farmers' markets. If you can't find them in these places, ask for them. Many stores will listen and respond. There are also some online resources that will help you find farmers directly; www.eatwild.com is a good starting point.

Tools of the Trade

Beyond knowing where to find naked food, there are a couple of tools that will make your shopping experience much smoother and more efficient.

The Shopping List

One of the best ways to make your shopping trip super speedy is to come prepared. The shopping list is an absolute must. Don't expect to wander into the market or store and figure out what you need when you get there. That's a sure way to buy stuff you don't need, to forget something essential, and to require a second trip to the store later on. (I can't tell you how many times I've had to learn this from frustrating experience.) Take the five minutes to think through what you need and write it down.

If you want to take your shopping list to a whole new level, organize it according to the general layout of the store. Produce goes together. Dairy and eggs should be in one part of your list, whole grains in another, and housecleaning products in another. This might sound a little excessively organized, and yeah, it's a little much. But it does make a difference and reduces the time you spend gazing at your list to make sure you've got everything on it.

Reusable Bags

If you're going to eat naked, you might as well live naked, making your shopping experience an eco-friendly one. Buying local, seasonal, organic food is a fantastic way to reduce your environmental footprint. Why go to that effort and then put all that delicious food in a plastic bag? Your reusable bag will give you even more reason to be proud of the way you eat. And that overstuffed bag of plastic bags you're keeping under the sink will gradually diminish down to nothing.

In Summary

Finding naked food doesn't have to be a chore, although it might mean shopping in a new store or making a weekend trip to the farmers' market. As with the other aspects of transitioning to a naked diet, take it step-by-step. You don't have to do it all overnight. Check out the different options that are available to you in your area, and go with the one that best suits your lifestyle, needs, and budget.

13

cook naked

Some of my fondest memories from when I was a child are those from time I spent in the kitchen. My parents were both busy professionals, so they weren't often around when it was time to make dinner. This left my nanny, Aileen, in charge of the task. Wanting to keep me entertained and involved, she decided we would put on a cooking show. She'd get me all set with my hands washed and my little apron tied, and then she'd make dinner, explaining each step to our imaginary audience. I'd stand proudly next to her on my stool as her assistant, handing her a spoon here, a zucchini there, feeling incredibly important and delighted to be part of this magical experience that culminated in a delicious meal.

I can't tell you what she made or if it was she who taught me how to chop a pepper, but I can attribute my total love for the process of making a home-cooked meal to those early experiences. My parents would arrive home at about the time dinner was ready, and we'd gather around the table, sharing stories of our day. Looking back, I realize how lucky I was and how precious these moments were. We cooked our own food and sat down to dinner together, all of us eating the same thing. This doesn't happen often anymore. Even for me, the resolute foodie and health nut, sometimes dinner feels more like an annoying chore than an opportunity for nourishment and connection. Is it possible for us to bring back the family meal, home-cooked and eaten together?

Cooking Helps You Get Naked

One of the best ways to ensure that you're eating naked is to prepare your food yourself. Cooking gives you total control of the ingredients and the food preparation, which will usually lead to far healthier meals. When we eat prepared food or out at restaurants, we relinquish much of that control. Who knows what goes into the food or how it was prepared?

I know, I know. You don't have time, there's not an extra minute in the day, and the last thing you need to add to your overstuffed schedule is endless time slaving in the kitchen over a hot stove.

I understand. I'm a busy person too, and while I do love to cook a complex meal every once in a while, that's the exception, not the rule. What I've learned is that cooking naked doesn't have to be complex, particularly time-consuming, or a lot of work. In fact, the essence of cooking naked is simplicity. It takes a little practice, but you can be efficient in the kitchen and you'll soon learn that preparing real, fresh food is not only better for you and your family, but it's also a lot of fun and absolutely delicious.

I've distilled what I've learned about preparing food into three basic principles:

- Keep it simple

- Be efficient

- Make it fun

KILL YOUR MICROWAVE

The microwave is one of those kitchen appliances that sounded too good to be true. What's happening to the food to make it heat up so fast? And why is it so ridiculously hot in the middle?

A microwave heats your food by using electromagnetic energy to create molecular friction, which both heats your food and changes its molecular shape. This means it actually changes the nature of the food and has a strong tendency to overcook it. As you've probably experienced, microwaves heat the food from the inside out, the reverse of how a stove, oven, grill, or fire would cook it. Several studies have shown that microwaved food loses a significantly higher proportion of antioxidants and vitamins, and its proteins can be negatively affected. This happens even if you're just heating up a dish that was previously cooked (Vallejo, Tomas-Barberan, and Garcia-Viguera 2003; Pitchford 2002).

Principle 1: Keep It Simple

Cooking naked is simple cooking. I'm not talking about gourmet cooking or a five-course meal. I'm not going to ask you to hunt down mysterious ingredients you've never heard of before. Cooking naked is taking the naked ingredients we looked at in the first part of this book and making meals out of a handful of them at a time. Nothing fancy, nothing complex, but *lots* of delicious flavor.

Few Ingredients

Tasty doesn't have to be complicated and involved. In fact, some of the simplest meals are some of the most delicious. I'm not going to give you an arbitrary cap on the number of ingredients to use, but know that you can make a delicious meal with just three or four main ingredients. If they're fresh and you have some good-quality fats to go along with them, all you need is a fresh herb or a squeeze of lemon or some freshly ground sea salt and pepper for the dish to come alive.

Let me give you an example. Today is the end of the week and there's little left in the fridge. Deadlines are looming and I've got no time to go shopping. Here's what I had to work with: a couple of eggs, some feta cheese, half a bag of salad greens, some spinach, a zucchini, three roasted beets, a couple of handfuls of cherry tomatoes, leftover cooked red quinoa, and a piece of salmon. With little effort, I turned those simple ingredients into three full, satisfying, nutritious meals that didn't take much time to prepare.

Breakfast was two eggs with zucchini and tomatoes scrambled lightly in organic butter. Lunch was a big salad using up the rest of the greens with red quinoa, some cherry tomatoes, crumbled feta cheese, and a few capers to add some zest. I topped the salad with a homemade dressing of olive oil, lemon juice, and a little mustard. For dinner, I had the salmon cooked in a little olive oil on a bed of spinach with some roasted beets and sautéed zucchini. Delicious, easy, and only four main ingredients. Each meal took around ten minutes to prepare.

Minimal Cooking

One of the tricks to simple cooking is minimal cooking. By that I mean eating some things raw and cooking others only lightly. Veggies

SNACKS are a great place to apply the principle of keeping it simple. They don't have to be fancy or involve much work. Here are a few ideas, designed to keep you going without overfilling you or slowing you down.

Kale chips: Deliciously crisp and a little salty, kale chips are an excellent replacement for potato chips, and very simple to make. Preheat the oven to 400°F. Take 1 bunch of kale, trim away the stems, and coarsely chop the leaves; you should have about 3 cups. Toss the kale with 1 tablespoon of extra-virgin olive oil until evenly coated, then spread it on a baking sheet and sprinkle with ¼ teaspoon of sea salt. Bake for 5 minutes, then stir and bake for another 5 to 6 minutes, until just brown and crispy.

Half avocado: Cut an avocado in half. Store the half with the pit for another time. Squeeze about ½ teaspoon of lemon or lime juice over and into the avocado, then sprinkle with a pinch of sea salt, and a pinch of chili powder if you like. Eat out of the shell with a spoon. What could be simpler?

Raw veggie sticks with hummus: If you have Classic Hummus (page 144) on hand, this snack is a no-brainer. Just slice various vegetables, such as carrot, celery, cucumber, bell pepper, and zucchini, into sticks and dip them into the hummus.

Fruit and nuts: Fruit is packed with vitamins, antioxidants, and other valuable nutrients, and its sugars give you quick energy, while the nuts provide good-quality fats and help moderate your blood sugar levels. A handful of nuts is the perfect amount to accompany a piece of fruit. I recommend that you soak and dry the nuts first (see chapter 9).

Hard-boiled eggs: If you're looking for perfect protein, this is the snack for you. Hard-boiled eggs are one of my favorite snacks. If I know I'm going to be on the run, I'll make several hard-boiled eggs at once and store them in the fridge for later in the week. For great results every time, try this method: Put the eggs in a single layer in a saucepan and add cold water to cover by at least an inch or two. Put the pan on the stove over medium heat to slowly bring the water to a boil. As soon as the water starts to boil, remove from the heat, cover the pot, and leave the eggs in the water for 10 to 12 minutes to finish cooking. Use a slotted spoon to transfer the eggs to a plate, then let them cool to room temperature. Hard-boiled eggs can be stored in the refrigerator for up to 5 days. Keep them in a covered container, or they might make your fridge a little smelly.

are perhaps the easiest to cook minimally. Raw veggies make excellent snacks and just need a wash and some creative slicing. Salads can be fast to prepare because there's usually no cooking involved. Lightly steamed or sautéed veggies also take little time. Yes, it takes time to wash and chop, but practice will help you cut that time down significantly. Meats can also be cooked lightly. If you're eating high-quality meat—naked meat—eating it a little "pink" is actually healthier and more nutritious.

The only exception to this rule is when it comes to grains. Grains need to be properly prepared, a lost tradition in our speed-driven society. Even though proper preparation of grains does take some time, the good news is a lot of that time doesn't require your actual presence. It just takes some planning and forethought. As we saw in chapter 9, all grains contain phytic acid, an enzyme inhibitor that prevents the grain's easy digestion and blocks the absorption of other important minerals. If I want to have properly prepared oatmeal for breakfast, I need to think about that the night before and put the water and the oats in the pot before going to bed. By morning, the soaking will have greatly reduced the amount of phytic acid in the oatmeal, and the cooking part of making the oatmeal takes very little time. I'll often turn the pot on low while I go take a shower, and when I'm all clean, my breakfast is waiting for me.

Minimal cooking has several benefits, the obvious one being it reduces the preparation time for your meals. Perhaps more importantly, it leaves much more nutrition in the food. Overcooking and overprocessing deplete food of much of its nutritional value. The best part is that minimal cooking often leaves in more of the flavor, too.

Principle 2: Be Efficient

Efficiency goes hand in hand with simplicity. To me, "efficient" means smart. It doesn't mean cutting corners. It means being aware of what needs to be done and doing it in a way that makes the most of limited resources, in particular time and money.

Planning Is Key

I will confess: I'm an incurable planner. While I do love spontaneity at times, my default setting is to plan. In some situations, this can be a liability. But I have to say, when it comes to cooking and food preparation, planning can be the difference between success and failure.

The first piece to plan is what you're going to eat in the next few days. You don't need to have every meal planned out; a couple of good ideas for one or two breakfasts, lunches, and dinners are enough to get you going. This will mean you're not scrambling to figure it out when you need to be making the food. You've done the thinking beforehand, and your task becomes simply preparation.

The next piece to plan is getting groceries. Enter the grocery list. I introduced this in chapter 12, so I don't need to say more here other than that I highly recommend making a list based on these meals *before* going shopping. Enough said.

I'm sure you've heard the advice to never grocery shop when you're hungry, and the same can be said for cooking. Shopping when you're hungry leads to poor decisions and often buying too much food. Have a small snack at home before you head out the door if you're at all peckish. Cooking when you're hungry is also a recipe for trouble, because you don't function well on no food, and it can be tempting to throw something together that's less nutritious simply because you've waited too long and now speed is your top priority.

Make It Once, Use It Lots

One of the best ways to make the fullest use of the time you spend in the kitchen—and thus to reduce the time you need to spend prepping your food—is to make lots of something that can be used throughout the week. Here are some examples.

Rice. If you're making a pot of rice, make a really big pot, more than you need for one meal. That way, you can use it in other ways throughout the week.

Dressings and sauces. Make two or three different dressings or sauces once, and use them in various ways throughout the week. This is an important part of eating naked because so many of the ingredients we want to avoid, like poor-quality fats, unnecessary extra sugars, and excessive sodium tend to find their way into commercial dressings and sauces. Making your own is the best way to ensure you're only getting the good stuff. Try out some of the recipes included later in this chapter.

Meat. Make extra meat for dinner and use it sliced, cold on a salad, or in a wrap with some veggies the next day for lunch. Sandwich and deli meats often are loaded with sodium, nitrates, and other preservatives best left out of our lunches. And really, some sliced flat-iron steak from last night's dinner over a salad is so much more delicious than salty sandwich meat.

Even better, bring back the Sunday night roast dinners. My grandmother used to do this every Sunday night. We'd have a big family dinner with a roast, lots of veggies, and a homemade pie for dessert. Yum! What I didn't realize until later was how strategic this was. She put lots of effort into one big meal on the weekend, when there was time to do so. She brought the whole family together every week to share in this ritual. *And,* she had leftovers she could use for the next few days for sandwiches, salads, and all sorts of creative things she came up with. Voilà! Her work in the kitchen was greatly reduced for the rest of the week.

More about leftovers. When you've got leftovers in the fridge, don't feel limited to an exact repeat of last night's dinner. Use elements of it in different ways. For example, you might have a quinoa salad as a side at dinner. The next day, you can put the leftovers of that salad along with some fresh lettuce and additional veggies into a wrap for lunch. I've been known to take veggies from last night's dinner and turn them into breakfast by poaching a couple of eggs and putting them on top.

I like to use these strategies as I go during the week. I make extra at each meal so that I can either repeat the meal or use parts of it in another one. I also like to have one day in the week as my primary food-prep day. I'll make a couple of dressings, maybe some hummus or a homemade salsa, a pot of rice, and some other basics that I'll use throughout the week. These are the most time-consuming parts of cooking, so I'll do them all at once, normally on a weekend after a trip to the farmers' market, and just have those foods in the fridge.

Have a Few Very Good Tools

Having good kitchen equipment will make your life in the kitchen far, far easier. You don't need to have a lot, just some basic essentials. My list of must-have kitchen tools includes the following.

- **One or two sharp knives:** Dull, crappy knives are the fastest way to slow you down and increase your risk of cutting yourself. The duller the knife, the harder you have to work. All you need are one or two good-quality knives that you keep sharp. Don't use them for anything except food preparation.

- **A salad spinner:** If you're buying fresh produce, in particular leafy greens, you'll need to wash and dry them. A salad spinner will make this task quick, easy, and clean.

- **A blender or food processor:** Salad dressings, sauces, homemade hummus, smoothies… These go from labor-intensive to easy-peasy with a blender or food processor.

- **A four-sided grater:** Each side has its own grate size and style, and you can do many things with it. Slice veggies in a hurry, grate some carrots to put on a salad, finely mince some ginger, and so on.

- **Food-storage containers of various sizes:** These go hand in hand with the "make it once, use it lots" guideline. The best containers are reusable, dishwasher safe, and ideally glass or ceramic so that you can throw them in the oven to reheat without having plastic leaching into your food. That said, hard plastic is fine, too, just don't heat the food in it (especially in the microwave, although you've already gotten rid of that by now).

EAT NAKED ON A BUDGET

I hear many arguments about whether cooking at home is cheaper than eating out. Clearly there are many factors: the quality of the restaurant, the quality of your food, if you're buying things when they're in or out of season, and how many people you're feeding. In my opinion, eating out is far more expensive than preparing food at home, particularly when you look at expenses beyond the simple cost of the food. Home-cooked meals are typically much healthier than restaurant or premade, simply for the fact that you're using higher-quality ingredients and not all that unhealthy industrial fat, excess salt, and sugar. Healthier meals lead to healthier people, which in and of itself lowers the cost of living. Save your restaurant dollars for a special occasion and cook at home.

- **A few good copper or stainless-steel pots**: One two-quart pot for grains and an eight-quart pot for soups and stock, a medium sauté pan, and one eight-inch or ten-inch skillet should suffice.

- **A steamer basket:** This is invaluable for veggie preparation. Just make sure that it fits the size of pot you have.

- **A flexible, heat-resistant spatula:** This will come in handy for sautéing veggies, flipping meats, and scraping out the sides of your food processor or blender when you're making a sauce or dressing.

Clean as You Go

One of the most daunting parts of home cooking can be the clean-up. I will admit it here publicly: I loathe doing dishes. It is by far my least favorite part of dealing with food. The day I acquired a dishwasher was a very happy day.

The way I make cleaning less overwhelming is to clean as I go. There isn't a meal I prepare where I'm not rinsing, tidying, wiping, and putting things into the dishwasher as I move through the meal preparation. This means that there's less to clean when dinner's over, and also that anything that could stick or require scrubbing is either already rinsed off or has had a chance to soak.

Another great strategy is to delegate who cooks and who cleans. It's house rules at our place that whoever makes dinner doesn't have to do dishes. That's probably another factor in my preference for being the chef of the house.

Principle 3: Make It Fun

My nanny Aileen's strategy of setting up a mock cooking show is a great example of the fun you can have with naked cooking. If you have kids, get them involved in making dinner. If you start them young, by the time they're teens you might have some budding chefs—or at least a pair of extra hands to take on food-preparation responsibilities a night or two a week. If you don't have kids, experiment to see how you can bring some

---

MY FAVORITE COOKING RITUALS

When it's time to prepare a meal, there are certain things I like to do:

- Put on my apron. There's something very sexy about a good apron, I think. Sometimes I'm inspired to put on heels as well, to make it even more special.

- Turn on my cooking tunes. These vary depending on my mood, from ambient jazz (dinnertime, especially on a weekend) to some of my favorite '80s tunes (weekend afternoon food prep for the week) to King's College Boys' Choir (Sunday morning brunch).

- If it's a weekend or the next day is a light one, I'll pour myself a glass of red wine. If it's a weeknight or I have an early morning, I'll pour myself a glass of mineral water with some lemon or, in the winter, have a cup of herbal tea.

- Kick everyone out of "my" side of the kitchen so I have room to move about quickly and freely without the risk of crashing into anyone.

- If it's wintertime and already dark outside, I'll light a candle or two to give the kitchen some added atmosphere.

With cooking, as with many things in life, what you put in is what you get out. This is a familiar idea in this book, especially with respect to the quality of your ingredients. This can be extended to your attitude when you walk into the kitchen. If you approach cooking expecting it to be hard, complicated, and generally a pain in the rear, then it will be. If you approach it as an adventure and a way to take some time to really nurture yourself, then it can be quite a pleasurable experience.

---

ritual to cooking. Light a candle, turn on some of your favorite music, maybe even pour yourself a glass of wine. Do something to make it less work and more play.

Make Mistakes

As a wise friend said to me, "A carrot is still a carrot, no matter how you slice it." Take this to heart in the kitchen. No one's expecting you to be a cordon bleu chef or to know how to make a perfect homemade soup the first time.

If you're like me (a bit of a perfectionist), this one can be tough. But, like me, you can learn to let that drive for perfection go. Make a mess of it the first time. It's difficult to make a meal truly inedible, and sometimes mistakes lead to really creative new dishes. At the very least, a kitchen disaster can be quite funny and make a great story later on. The only way to learn to cook is to try, so go ahead and botch your first salad dressing. Before long, cooking will be second nature and you'll wonder what the big deal was.

Naked Recipes

Now that we've looked at how to get naked in the kitchen, let's move on to some recipe ideas. The most important thing about cooking naked is to get out there and try it. With the help of the wonderful chef James Barry, I've included some of my favorite recipes here, along with some new creations we concocted together.

We've designed these recipes to complement each other. For example, the pesto in the "Basics" section is used in one of the salad recipes. You can use the bones from the Easy Roast Chicken (page 160) in the Chicken Stock (page 138), which makes a great base for several of the soups. Have a look through the recipes and start with whatever calls to you.

Most of these recipes are free of gluten and soy, and exceptions are noted. Also, for those with food sensitivities, we've made sure there are alternates in each food category that don't include some of the primary allergens, such as dairy, eggs, and nuts.

Introducing the Chef

Through a chance encounter earlier this year, I met the incredibly talented chef James Barry, who shares with me a passion for truly scrumptious naked foods. A graduate of the Natural Gourmet Institute for Health and Culinary Arts in New York, James has worked as a private chef for many clients, including several celebrities, and now leads his company Wholesome2go, a healthy, high-quality food delivery company. James was a crucial part of the development of the recipes that follow. Many of them are his creations, and all of them have been greatly improved by his tips to take them over the top. Enjoy!

Basics

The basics in this section are things that are useful to have around, and that you can use in a variety of ways. The kitchen standards that you'll find in this section are also called for in recipes in other sections of this chapter.

CHICKEN STOCK

Makes 1 to 2 quarts

One of the best parts of roast chicken is the yummy chicken stock you can make with the bones. After your chicken dinner, remove any chicken from the bones and store it in a sealed container in the fridge for later. For example, you can add it to the Mixed Green Salad recipe on page 144 for a tasty lunch, and use the bones as described below to make a scrumptious chicken stock.

What's great about stocks is that it doesn't matter how you cut the veggies that go into them, and you can use all the parts of the vegetables, even the "ugly" bits that you'd normally discard. You can even throw in the celery leaves and the little green bit at the top of the carrots, and you don't need to peel the carrots. Just make sure that everything you put in the stock is dirt free and you're good to go. Even though it takes a long time to cook, it's not something you need to babysit. And the fragrances wafting from the kitchen while you're cooking are worth every minute of effort that goes into it.

Be sure to use a mild vinegar, such as white vinegar, apple cider vinegar, or red or white wine vinegar. The main purpose of the vinegar isn't for flavoring; it's to help pull the minerals out of the bones, so it's very important to include it. Note that the yield of this recipe depends on the size of the pot you use. In a larger pot, you'll need to add more water to cover the ingredients, so you'll end up with more stock, whereas a smaller pot will yield less stock, but the flavor may be richer.

1 stripped chicken carcass, plus any organ parts

1 onion, coarsely chopped

2 carrots, coarsely chopped

2 stalks celery, coarsely chopped

1 jalapeño pepper, coarsely chopped (leave the seeds in for a spicier flavor)

2 bay leaves

1 teaspoon mild vinegar

Put the chicken carcass and any organ parts into an 8-quart soup pot, along with the onion, carrots, celery, jalapeño, bay leaves, and vinegar. Add enough filtered water to just cover everything (about 3 quarts). Cover and bring to a boil over high heat.

Once the stock is boiling, turn the heat down as low as possible, skim off any scum that has risen to the top, and let simmer uncovered for 8 to 12 hours.

Let the stock cool for about 30 minutes. Strain the stock through a fine-mesh sieve and discard the bones and veggies.

If using the stock within a few days, store it in the fridge. Otherwise, store it in ziplock freezer bags in the freezer for up to 3 months. If the stock is still warm when you put it in the fridge, leave it uncovered until it's fully cooled. Covering it will keep it warm longer, creating a breeding ground for bacteria.

Tip from Chef James: You can freeze stock in an ice cube tray to make it easier to thaw just the portion you need. Once the stock has frozen, transfer the cubes to a freezer bag. Just grab as many cubes as you need instead of using commercially made broths or bouillon cubes, which are often jam-packed with preservatives and synthetic flavor enhancers.

Veggie Stock Variation

If you're a vegetarian and don't want to use a chicken carcass for your stock, you can replace it with a handful of eggshells, leaving everything else the same. The eggshells will provide some of the minerals that you'd otherwise get from the chicken carcass.

BALSAMIC VINAIGRETTE

Makes about 1 cup

You'll notice this recipe calls for Dijon mustard, which is a packaged food. You can make your own mustard, but for this purpose, a premade mustard that uses real, naked ingredients is fine. Read the label to make sure you recognize all the ingredients and that there's no added sugar.

¼ cup balsamic vinegar

1 tablespoon Dijon mustard

½ teaspoon sea salt

½ teaspoon freshly ground black pepper

2 tablespoons chopped fresh basil, or 1 teaspoon dried

1 clove garlic

¾ cup extra-virgin olive oil

Combine the vinegar, mustard, salt, pepper, basil, and garlic in a blender or food processor and blend until smooth. With the motor running, slowly drizzle in the oil and continue blending until smooth.

Tip from Chef James: To make this dressing creamy and a little cheesy, add ¼ cup of any soft cheese (mascarpone, cream cheese, ricotta, chèvre, and so on) at the end and blend until smooth.

CREAMY GINGER DRESSING

Makes 1½ cups

I recommend that you always choose tamari, rather than commercial soy sauce. It's a fermented product, made using traditional methods, whereas soy sauce is made using an industrial processing method that damages the integrity of the soy. If gluten is an issue, be sure to use a wheat-free soy sauce.

- 1 tablespoon Dijon mustard
- ¼ cup apple cider vinegar
- 3 tablespoons tamari
- 1 tablespoon white miso
- 1 small carrot, coarsely chopped
- 1 teaspoon grated ginger
- 3 pitted dates
- 2 tablespoons tahini
- ¾ cup raw sesame oil

Combine the mustard, vinegar, tamari, miso, carrot, ginger, dates, and tahini in a blender or food processor and blend until smooth. With the motor running, slowly drizzle in the oil and continue blending until smooth.

Tip from Chef James: If you freeze ginger, it's much easier to grate.

SALSA

Makes 1 cup of smooth salsa, or 1½ cups if left chunky

1 small carrot, coarsely chopped

2 cloves garlic, coarsely chopped

1 jalapeño pepper, coarsely chopped (leave the seeds in for a
  spicier flavor)

½ cup packed cilantro

Juice of ½ lime

3 tomatoes, coarsely chopped

½ teaspoon sea salt

Put all of the ingredients in a food processor or blender and pulse lightly
for a chunky salsa, or process until smooth. If you like your salsa less
watery, after processing drain the salsa through a strainer to remove
any excess liquid.

PESTO

Makes ½ cup

There are endless ways to use pesto. Try it on roasted vegetables, as a marinade for meat, with your eggs in the morning, or in the Pesto Romaine Salad (page 146). In the summertime, when basil is fresh and abundant, pesto is a favorite at my house. It's easy to modify this recipe to accommodate any food allergies. If dairy is an issue, replace the Parmesan cheese with 2 teaspoons of mellow white miso, and if nuts are an issue, use pumpkin seeds rather than pine nuts. Or if nuts aren't a problem but pine nuts are too pricey, this pesto also tastes great with walnuts.

¼ cup pine nuts, pumpkin seeds, or walnuts

2 cloves garlic

1 cup packed fresh basil

¼ cup extra-virgin olive oil

1 cup packed fresh spinach

1 tablespoon grated Parmesan cheese, or 2 teaspoons mellow white miso

½ teaspoon sea salt

Pinch of freshly ground black pepper

Put the pine nuts, garlic, and basil in a food processor or blender and process until finely chopped. With the motor running, slowly drizzle in the oil. Add the spinach and process until incorporated, scraping down the sides if need be. Add the Parmesan, salt, and pepper, and process until it forms a paste. This pesto stores well in the fridge for up to 1 week. You can also make multiple batches and freeze the pesto in an ice cube tray, although this might affect the color.

Tip from Chef James: To take this pesto over the top, add ¼ teaspoon of lemon zest when you add the Parmesan, salt, and pepper. The lemon brings out the other flavors and adds a beautifully subtle zing to the pesto.

CLASSIC HUMMUS

Makes 1½ cups

When purchasing any type of canned beans, watch out for high levels of sodium. Read the label and get the lowest-sodium brand you can find. This recipe calls for about ¼ cup of liquid, as needed to achieve the consistency you prefer. If you're using home-cooked beans, you can use some of the cooking liquid, and if using canned beans, just use water. Vegetable stock would also be fine.

> 1½ cups soaked and cooked garbanzo beans, or 1 (15-ounce) can, well rinsed
>
> 2 tablespoons freshly squeezed lemon juice (about ½ lemon)
>
> 1 clove garlic
>
> 2 tablespoons tahini
>
> ½ teaspoon ground cumin
>
> Pinch of cayenne pepper
>
> ½ teaspoon sea salt
>
> 1 tablespoon extra-virgin olive oil
>
> ¼ cup water or other liquid

Put the garbanzo beans, lemon juice, garlic, tahini, cumin, cayenne, and salt in a blender or food processor and blend until smooth. With the motor running, slowly drizzle in the oil, then add the water as necessary to achieve the desired consistency.

Variation

Add ¼ cup packed fresh basil and ¼ cup coarsely chopped sun-dried tomatoes to the base before adding the oil.

Salads and Sides

The following salads and sides can be used to complement a larger meal or, if you add a little protein, as a main course.

RAW CAULIFLOWER "COUSCOUS"

Serves 3 or 4

This raw cauliflower salad is a great substitute for couscous dishes. It's far more nutritious, and it's gluten free. It's also super easy to make—if you have a food processor. If you don't, I recommend that you skip this recipe. Chopping the cauliflower so finely without the help of a food processor would just be too much work.

1 cauliflower

¼ cup finely chopped red bell pepper

¼ cup chopped tomato

¼ cup packed fresh parsley

1 tablespoon packed fresh mint

½ clove garlic

½ teaspoon grated lemon zest

¼ teaspoon paprika

¼ teaspoon ground cumin

½ teaspoon sea salt

2 tablespoons walnut oil

1 tablespoon freshly squeezed lemon juice

Rinse the cauliflower, cut it into quarters and trim the stem. Coarsely chop the cauliflower, then put it in a food processor and grind it until it has a fine consistency similar to couscous.

Transfer the cauliflower to a large bowl (no need to clean the processor just yet). Stir in the bell pepper and tomato.

Put the parsley, mint, and garlic in the food processor and process until finely chopped. Add the mixture to the cauliflower, along with the lemon zest, paprika, cumin, salt, oil, and lemon juice. Mix well. Refrigerate until well chilled before serving.

PESTO ROMAINE SALAD

Serves 4

1 head romaine lettuce, washed and torn or chopped into small pieces

1 avocado, chopped

½ cucumber, peeled and chopped

Handful of sunflower or other sprouts

3 tablespoons Pesto (page 143)

¼ cup cubed fresh mozzarella cheese

Combine the lettuce, avocado, cucumber, and sprouts in a large salad bowl. Toss with the pesto and cheese, and enjoy!

MIXED GREEN SALAD

Serves 4

I have to admit that I'm a fan of packaged salad greens. Although the packaging is a downside, it can be recycled in many communities, and the prewashed greens really cut down on preparation time. You may also be able to find high-quality baby salad greens in bulk.

5 ounces mixed baby greens

1 medium carrot, grated (about ½ cup)

1 medium beet, peeled and grated (about 1 cup)

½ cup diced green bell pepper

¼ cup crumbled feta cheese

½ cup loosely packed sprouts, any kind

1 tablespoon finely chopped green onion

¼ cup chopped walnuts

½ cup Balsamic Vinaigrette (page 140)

Combine the greens, carrot, beet, and bell pepper in a large salad bowl. Sprinkle the feta cheese, sprouts, green onion, and walnuts over the top, then drizzle on the vinaigrette and serve right away. (Most lettuce will lose its crispness the longer it sits in a dressing, so it's always a good idea to eat a green salad immediately after you dress it.)

ASPARAGUS WITH BUTTER MUSHROOMS

Serves 4

This is an easy and absolutely delicious way to prepare asparagus, and it makes a great side for the Seared Salmon (page 164). Remember to use asparagus when it's fresh and in season, in springtime.

> 1 tablespoon butter
>
> 1 cup thinly sliced cremini mushrooms
>
> Pinch of sea salt
>
> 1 bunch asparagus, bottoms chopped off
>
> Pinch of red pepper flakes (optional)
>
> ½ teaspoon grated lemon zest (optional)

Heat the butter in a small skillet over medium heat. Add the mushrooms and salt and sauté for 4 to 5 minutes, until tender and lightly browned.

Meanwhile, set up a steamer and bring the water to a boil. Steam the asparagus for 2 to 3 minutes, being careful not to overcook it; it should still be slightly crisp. Transfer the asparagus to a cold plate so it doesn't continue to cook.

Scatter the mushrooms over the asparagus, then sprinkle with the red pepper flakes and lemon zest.

Tip from Chef James: To save time when preparing the asparagus, test one piece to determine the breaking point, and then chop all the bottoms off at once, with the asparagus still bundled together.

SPICY GARLIC GREEN BEANS

Serves 2

I've never been a huge fan of green beans, probably because I ate so many stringy canned beans as a kid. They've always seemed particularly bland and boring to me, so I've often skipped past them at the market—until now. This recipe is so easy and flavorful it has converted me into a green bean lover. Curry powder and chili powder are both blended spices, so un-naked ingredients can sneak in unnoticed if you're not careful. Look for organic brands that don't have ingredients you can't pronounce, excessive salt, sugar, or MSG.

- 1 tablespoon coconut oil
- ½ teaspoon curry powder
- ¼ teaspoon chili powder
- ½ teaspoon sea salt
- Pinch of freshly ground black pepper
- 8 ounces green beans, ends trimmed
- 2 cloves garlic, thinly sliced

Preheat the oven to 375°F.

Put the oil, curry powder, chili powder, salt, and pepper in a large bowl and stir them together. (If the coconut oil is solid, which it will be if your kitchen is a little cool, put it in a stainless steel mixing bowl and pop it in the oven for 30 to 60 seconds as the oven is warming. The oil will melt very quickly.)

Add the beans and garlic and toss with the oil and spices until evenly coated. Spread the beans in an even layer on a baking sheet.

Bake for 5 minutes, then turn the beans and bake for another 5 minutes, until slightly browned. If you like your beans wilted, extend the cooking times to 10 minutes on each side.

GARLIC BROCCOLI RABE AND SUMMER SQUASH

Serves 4

This dish is a great accompaniment for Seared Salmon (page 164) or Easy Roasted Chicken (page 158).

> 1 teaspoon coconut oil
>
> 3 cloves garlic, thinly sliced
>
> 1 small crookneck yellow squash, cut into half-moons
>
> 1 bunch broccoli rabe, coarsely chopped (about 3 cups, firmly packed)
>
> ¼ teaspoon sea salt
>
> ¼ teaspoon red pepper flakes (optional)

Heat the oil in large skillet over medium heat. Add the garlic and sauté for 2 minutes. Add the squash and sauté for 2 more minutes. Add the broccoli rabe and stir until everything is thoroughly combined.

Cover and cook for 2 minutes, just until the broccoli rabe is bright green. Sprinkle with the salt and red pepper flakes and serve warm.

Tip: It's okay if the broccoli rabe still has a little water on it after rinsing. This will help to steam it.

ASIAN NOODLE SALAD

Serves 4

This salad makes delicious use of the Creamy Ginger Dressing (page 141). In terms of noodles, my personal preference is mung bean noodles (sometimes called glass noodles). If these aren't readily available, try soba or brown rice vermicelli. If you add some tempeh or leftover chicken or shrimp, this becomes a delicious and filling meal. I recommend low-sodium, wheat-free tamari.

- 6 ounces Asian-style noodles
- 2 tablespoons coconut oil
- 6 large shiitake mushrooms, stemmed and thinly sliced (about 1 cup)
- 2 tablespoons tamari
- 2 cups finely chopped Napa cabbage
- 2 small carrots, grated
- 1 cucumber, thinly sliced into half-moons
- ¼ cup finely chopped snow peas
- 2 cups fresh baby spinach leaves
- 2 green onions, finely chopped (about 2 teaspoons)
- ½ cup Creamy Ginger Dressing (page 141)
- 2 teaspoons sesame seeds

Fill a large saucepan three-quarters full with water. Bring the water to a boil, then add the noodles and cook until al dente. (If using packaged noodles, follow the instructions on the package. Some Asian noodles are soaked in hot water, not boiled.) Drain the noodles.

Meanwhile, heat the oil in small skillet over medium heat. Add the mushrooms and sauté for about 5 minutes, until tender. Add the tamari, stir to coat the mushrooms, and immediately remove from the heat.

Transfer the mushrooms to a large bowl. Add the cabbage, carrots, cucumber, snow peas, spinach, green onions, noodles, and dressing. Toss until well combined. Sprinkle the sesame seeds over the salad and enjoy!

Soups

Soups make great lunches and dinners, as sides or main dishes, for any time of the year. We've included a chilled gazpacho for summer, along with several winter favorites.

SUMMER GAZPACHO

Serves 4

Chopping all of the vegetables for this soup can be a little time-consuming. To save time, you can chop the bell peppers, jalapeño, onion, garlic, and parsley in a food processor.

- ½ small yellow bell pepper, finely chopped (about ½ cup)
- ½ small red bell pepper, finely chopped (about ½ cup)
- 1 jalapeño pepper, finely chopped (leave the seeds in for a spicier flavor)
- ¼ small red onion, finely chopped (about ¼ cup)
- 2 small cloves garlic, minced
- 1 teaspoon minced fresh parsley
- 2 cups canned tomatoes
- 1 tablespoon freshly squeezed lemon juice
- 1 teaspoon sea salt
- 1 avocado, diced
- 1 cup soaked and cooked garbanzo beans, or 1 cup canned, well rinsed

Put the bell peppers, jalapeño, onion, garlic, and parsley in a bowl.

Puree the tomatoes in a blender or food processor, then add them to the bowl of veggies. Add the lemon juice, salt, avocado, and garbanzo beans and stir until well combined.

You can serve the gazpacho immediately, or refrigerate until chilled. It's best when it's been refrigerated overnight, as this allows the flavors to meld nicely.

VEGGIE BEAN SOUP

Serves 6

This is a light soup I like to pair with a salad when I don't need a big meal to feel satisfied. Use your favorite white bean in this recipe: great northern beans, white kidney beans, navy beans, or white adzuki beans.

1 tablespoon extra-virgin olive oil

½ cup finely diced onion

Sea salt

2 stalks celery, finely diced (about 1 cup)

2 carrots, finely diced or grated (about 1 cup)

1 medium tomato, finely diced (about ½ cup)

1 bay leaf

1 jalapeño pepper, finely diced (leave the seeds in for a spicier flavor)

1 medium zucchini, grated (about 1 cup)

1½ cups soaked and cooked white beans, or 1 (15-ounce) can of white beans, well rinsed

1 teaspoon dried oregano

2 cups Chicken Stock (page 138) or Veggie Stock (see page 139)

2 cups packed fresh spinach

Freshly ground black pepper

Heat the oil in a large saucepan over medium heat. Add the onion and a pinch of salt and sauté for 2 minutes. Add the celery and sauté for 2 more minutes. Add the carrots and another pinch of salt and sauté for 2 more minutes. Stir in the tomato, bay leaf, jalapeño, zucchini, and beans, then stir in the oregano and stock. Turn the heat up to high, cover, and bring to a boil.

Lower the heat and simmer, uncovered, for 10 minutes, until the vegetables are tender.

Remove from the heat, add the spinach, and cover. Let stand for about 3 minutes, until the spinach has wilted a bit. Season with black pepper to taste and serve warm.

ROASTED ROOT SOUP

Serves 4

- ½ kabocha or large acorn squash
- 1 teaspoon plus 1 tablespoon coconut oil
- 2 large carrots, coarsely chopped (about 2 cups)
- 1 medium onion, coarsely chopped (about 1½ cups)
- 1 large parsnip, coarsely chopped (about 1½ cups)
- 4 cloves garlic, peeled
- 3 cups Chicken Stock (page 138) or Veggie Stock (see page 139)
- 1¼ teaspoons sea salt
- 2 teaspoons freshly squeezed lemon juice
- 1 tablespoon finely chopped fresh parsley (optional)

Preheat the oven to 385°F.

Cut the squash in half lengthwise, leaving the seeds in. Rub the cut sides of the squash with the 1 teaspoon coconut oil. Put the squash halves on a baking sheet cut side down and bake for 20 to 25 minutes, until slightly squishy when pinched.

Meanwhile, toss the carrots, onion, parsnip, and garlic with the 1 table-spoon coconut oil, then spread them on another baking sheet in an even layer. (If the coconut oil is solid, which it will be if your kitchen is a little cool, put it in a stainless steel mixing bowl and pop it into the oven for 30 to 60 seconds. The oil will melt quickly.) Bake for 15 minutes, then turn the veggies and bake for 10 more minutes.

Let the squash stand until cool enough to handle. Scoop out the seeds with a large spoon, then scoop out the flesh and put it in a blender or food processor. You should have 1 to 1½ cups of squash flesh.

Add the roasted veggies and stock. Don't overfill the blender or the soup won't blend well. About halfway to three-quarters full is good, so you may need to work in batches. Puree the soup, removing the little center piece of the blender lid (to let the steam out) and using a towel to cover the hole and hold the lid down while you're blending (the combination of hot liquid and blending can make the lid pop off).

Pour the soup into a serving bowl, then stir in the salt and lemon juice. Garnish with the parsley and serve warm.

BROCCOLI SOUP

Serves 4

---

2 teaspoons extra-virgin olive oil

1 onion, coarsely chopped (about 2 cups)

2 cloves garlic, coarsely chopped

1 large potato (red or russet), coarsely chopped

2 cups Chicken Stock (page 138) or Veggie Stock (see page 139)

1 sprig of fresh rosemary

½ teaspoon sea salt

4 cups coarsely chopped broccoli (about 1 bunch)

About ½ teaspoon freshly squeezed lemon juice

Heat the oil in a large saucepan over medium heat. Add the onion and garlic and sauté for 2 to 3 minutes, until soft. Stir in the potato, stock, rosemary, and salt. Cover and bring to a boil, then lower the heat and simmer for 15 minutes.

Add the broccoli and simmer for 10 minutes, making sure not to overcook the broccoli (bright green is good; pale green means it's overcooked).

Transfer the mixture to a blender or food processor. Don't overfill the blender or the soup won't blend well; about halfway to three-quarters full is good, so you may need to work in batches. Puree the soup until smooth and creamy, removing the little center piece of the blender lid (to let the steam out) and using a towel to cover the hole and hold the lid down while you're blending (the combination of hot liquid and blending can make the lid pop off). Stir in the lemon juice, adjusting the amount as desired. Enjoy!

THAI CHICKEN SOUP

Serves 4

This soothing soup is a favorite around our house, especially during cold season. For a vegetarian version, replace the chicken stock with veggie stock and replace the cooked chicken with 1 cup cooked quinoa. As always, I recommend tamari over commercial soy sauce, preferably a low-sodium, wheat-free variety of tamari.

- 2 teaspoons coconut oil
- 4 shiitake mushrooms, thinly sliced
- 2 cloves garlic, minced
- 2 small carrots, grated
- ¼ cup sliced red bell pepper, in ½-inch strips
- 2 teaspoons grated ginger (see Tip on page 141)
- 2 tablespoons tamari
- 2 cups Chicken Stock (page 138)
- 2 cups coconut milk
- 2 tablespoons freshly squeezed lime juice (about 1 lime)
- 1 cup shredded cooked chicken
- Small handful of snow peas, thinly sliced
- ½ teaspoon red pepper flakes (optional)

Heat the oil in a medium saucepan over medium heat. Add the mushrooms and garlic and sauté for 2 minutes. Add the carrots, bell pepper, and ginger and sauté for 2 more minutes. Add the tamari, stir to coat the vegetables, then immediately stir in the stock.

Cover, bring to a boil, then immediately turn the heat down to low. Stir in the coconut milk and lime juice and simmer, covered, for a few more minutes. Add the chicken and simmer, covered, for another 2 minutes, until the chicken is heated through.

Remove from the heat, add the snow peas and red pepper flakes, and let stand, covered, for 4 minutes. Serve warm and savor the soul-soothing properties of this delicious soup.

Entrées

Most of the entrées we've included here are a little more involved than the recipes in some of the other sections. These are great weekend meals, perfect for when you've got a little extra time to play in the kitchen.

LEMON AND ASPARAGUS RISOTTO

Serves 6

This is one of my favorite comfort-food dishes. Make it in spring when asparagus is in season. It's absolutely delicious paired with a salad, like the Mixed Green Salad (page 146). Arborio rice, an Italian variety of rice, is used to make risotto because it's particularly starchy. When it's cooked slowly, the starches release to create a nice, creamy consistency. It's a whole grain but has that texture of some of my favorite comfort foods. This dish is a bit time-consuming, but well worth the time and effort. It's a good thing to make when you're doing other kitchen tasks, as you do need to hover.

5 cups Chicken Stock (page 138) or Veggie Stock (see page 139)

2 tablespoons butter or extra-virgin olive oil

¼ cup finely minced onion

2 cloves garlic, thinly sliced

2 cups Arborio rice

2 cups cut asparagus, in ½-inch pieces

2 tablespoons chopped fresh dill, or 2 teaspoons dried

½ teaspoon grated lemon zest

2 tablespoons freshly squeezed lemon juice (about ½ lemon)

1 cup crumbled feta cheese

Put the stock in a medium saucepan over medium heat.

In a separate large saucepan, heat the butter over medium heat. Add the onion and garlic and sauté for 2 to 3 minutes, until the onion is translucent.

Turn the heat down to low, add the rice to the pan with the onions and garlic, and stir frequently for 2 minutes, making sure that all of the grains are coated with butter.

Add about ¾ cup of the stock and stir into the rice mixture. Once the liquid is absorbed, add another ¾ cup or so of stock. Continue in this way, adding stock and letting rice simmer, stirring occasionally, until the stock is absorbed. When only about 1 cup of the stock is left, gently stir in the asparagus, then add the remainder of the stock.

When all the stock has been absorbed into the rice, add the dill, lemon zest and juice, and feta cheese. Stir until the cheese has melted, about 2 minutes. Serve hot.

TORTILLA-LESS GREEN ENCHILADAS

Serves 4 to 6

This recipe ups the veggie factor by using collard green leaves, rather than tortillas, to wrap the fillings. For a video of how to assemble these unusual but delicious enchiladas, check my website (www.eatnakednow.com). For some flavor variety, try different peppers. We've suggested a pasilla or jalapeño, but you can also use poblano, serrano, or Anaheim. The general rule of thumb when it comes to peppers is the smaller the spicier. This recipe contains chile powder, which is a blended spice, so un-naked ingredients can sneak in unnoticed if you're not careful. Look for an organic brand that doesn't have ingredients you can't pronounce, excessive salt, sugar, or MSG.

> 1½ cups Chicken Stock (page 138), Veggie Stock (see page 139), or filtered water
>
> 1 cup brown basmati rice
>
> 2 tablespoons extra-virgin olive oil
>
> ½ cup diced onion
>
> 2 cloves garlic, minced
>
> ½ cup diced red bell pepper
>
> ½ cup diced yellow bell pepper
>
> 4 stalks celery, diced (about 1 cup)
>
> 1 carrot, grated (about ¼ cup)
>
> 4 cups coarsely chopped cauliflower
>
> 1 pasilla pepper or jalapeño pepper, finely diced (leave the seeds in for a spicier flavor)
>
> 1 cup diced zucchini
>
> 1 teaspoon chili powder
>
> 1 teaspoon ground cumin
>
> 1 big bunch of collard greens
>
> 1 cup soaked and cooked black beans, or 1 cup canned, well rinsed
>
> 1 cup grated Monterey Jack or mild Cheddar cheese (optional)

Put the stock in small saucepan, cover, and bring to a boil. Add the rice, cover, and bring back to a boil. Lower the heat and simmer until all of the liquid is absorbed, about 20 minutes.

Meanwhile, heat the oil in a large skillet over medium heat. Add the onion and sauté for 2 minutes. Add the garlic, bell peppers, celery, and carrot and sauté for 3 to 4 minutes.

Put the cauliflower and pasilla in a food processor and pulse until finely minced; if you don't have a food processor, you can mince them by hand. Add the cauliflower mixture to the skillet and sauté for 2 minutes. Add the zucchini last so it doesn't get too soft, and sauté for 2 more minutes. Stir in the chili powder and cumin and remove from the heat.

Set up a steamer and bring the water to a boil. Place the collard greens flat on a cutting board with their stems toward you. Cut off the stems and the bottom center part of the collard greens, cutting away an upside-down V-shaped section at the base of the leaves. Steam the collard greens for 3 to 4 minutes, until soft.

Mix the rice and beans together in a medium bowl.

To assemble the enchiladas, lay out a collard leaf with its backside facing up. Spread about ½ cup of the vegetable mixture across the lower third of leaf, then spread about ¼ cup of the rice mixture and 1 tablespoon of the cheese over the veggies. You may need to adjust the quantities somewhat based on the size of the leaf.

Starting at the bottom, fold the bottom edge of the leaf up and over the fillings. Fold both sides in, then roll up the enchilada. Serve right away. You can cut each enchilada in half crosswise for presentation if you like.

EASY ROAST CHICKEN

Serves 4 to 6

This recipe is a slight variation of the classic, inspired by Sunday dinners at my Gramma's house. I'm not a fan of dry chicken, and this recipe is guaranteed to give you nice juicy, tender chicken. Serve it with some roasted veggies and a salad one night, and then use the leftovers in a salad within a couple of days. And don't throw those bones away! Use the carcass to make Chicken Stock (page 138), which can then be used as a base for the Thai Chicken Soup (page 155). Now that's an efficient use of a chicken! For a naked white wine, choose an organic variety, and if you live in a region where wine is made, choose one from a vineyard close to you.

1 whole chicken (3 to 4 pounds)

Sea salt

1 lemon, quartered

1 head garlic, separated into cloves and peeled

4 sprigs of fresh rosemary

1 leek, halved lengthwise and sliced ½ inch thick, or 2 small onions, coarsely chopped

2 medium carrots, sliced ½ inch thick

1 cup dry white wine

About 1 cup filtered water

1 tablespoon butter

Freshly ground black pepper

Preheat the oven to 350°F.

Wash the chicken and pat with a paper towel to dry. Sprinkle the inside with salt, then stuff the chicken with half of the lemon wedges, half of the garlic cloves, and the rosemary.

Place the chicken in the middle of roasting pan (a large ceramic casserole dish works really well if you don't have a roasting pan, and I've even used a lasagna pan in a pinch). Arrange the leeks and carrots around the chicken, along with the remaining lemon wedges and garlic cloves. Add the wine and enough water to bring the liquid about ½ inch up the side of the pan.

Smear the butter on the chicken, then sprinkle liberally with salt and
pepper. Cover the pan (if the pan you're using doesn't have a lid, alu-
minum foil is fine). Bake for 1½ hours.

Remove the lid, baste the chicken with the juices, and bake uncovered for
another 15 to 20 minutes, until nicely browned.

Tip from Chef James: You can make a delicious and easy gravy
with the drippings from the chicken. Start by removing the lemon
wedges from the pan and discarding, then transfer the leek and
carrots to a serving dish. Add a tablespoon or two of flour to the pan
or, for a gluten-free gravy, add arrowroot powder (similar to cornstarch but much less processed) to the drippings and whisk together
over low heat until the gravy thickens. You can leave the garlic cloves
whole, or consider blending them into the gravy using a handheld
blender or food processor. This is a delicious topping for both the
roasted veggies and the chicken.

SMOKY LAMB RAGOUT ON SPAGHETTI SQUASH

Serves 4

This is a delicious wintertime recipe that will nourish you body and soul. The richness of the lamb and the smokiness of the chipotle pepper complement the subtleties of the spaghetti squash. The dish is a great whole-foods substitute for traditional spaghetti and meatballs—without the spaghetti and with a fragrant and innovative sauce. The cooking time is long (6 hours), making it a great weekend dinner.

Granulated onion and granulated garlic may not seem like the most naked of ingredients. However, they're simply dried onion and dried garlic that have been coarsely ground—unlike garlic and onion powder, which are ground more finely and often include anticaking agents and artificial ingredients. You'll find granulated onion and garlic in the spice section of your market. Both are good options for adding a lot of flavor without the bulk of fresh onions and garlic. For a naked red wine, choose an organic variety, and if you live in a region where wine is made, choose one from a vineyard close to you.

1 teaspoon chili powder

1 teaspoon paprika

½ teaspoon oregano

½ teaspoon granulated onion

½ teaspoon granulated garlic

½ teaspoon sea salt

3 teaspoons extra-virgin olive oil

1 lamb shank (about 1 pound)

½ cup chopped onion

2 cloves garlic, crushed

½ cup chopped green bell pepper

½ cup chopped red bell pepper

½ cup chopped celery

½ jalapeño pepper, finely chopped (leave the seeds in for a spicier flavor)

½ cup chopped cremini mushrooms

1 (28-ounce) can diced or crushed tomatoes

1 cup red wine

2 cups filtered water or Veggie Stock (see page 139)

1 bay leaf

1 dried chipotle pepper or other dried chile

1 large spaghetti squash

Freshly ground black pepper

1 cup finely chopped kale

1 tablespoon finely chopped parsley

Mix the chili powder, paprika, oregano, granulated onion, granulated garlic, and salt in a large bowl. Roll the lamb shank in the spice mix until evenly coated.

Pour 1 teaspoon of the olive oil into a pot large enough to fit the shank easily, and place it over medium heat. Add the lamb and cook until browned on all sides, about 2 minutes per side. Pull the shank out of the pan and set it aside.

Pour another teaspoon of the olive oil into the pan, then add the onion and garlic and sauté for 2 minutes. Add the bell peppers, celery, and jalapeño and sauté for 2 minutes. Add the mushrooms and sauté for 2 more minutes. Add the lamb, tomatoes, wine, water, bay leaf, and chipotle. Cover and bring to a boil.

Remove the lid, turn the heat down as low as possible, and simmer for about 6 hours, until the lamb is easily pulled off the bone.

About 45 minutes before the lamb is done, cook the spaghetti squash. Preheat the oven to 385°F. Cut the squash in half lengthwise (see Tip on page 162). Rub the cut sides of the squash with the remaining teaspoon of olive oil, then put the squash on a baking sheet cut side down and bake for 20 to 25 minutes, until the shell is soft when you gently press it. Let the squash stand until cool enough to handle.

Scoop out the squash seeds and discard them. Using a fork, scrape the flesh of the squash lengthwise, pulling it into spaghetti-like strings. Scoop the flesh into a serving dish or bowls and sprinkle with a pinch of salt and pepper.

continued

Pull the lamb shank out of the ragout. The flesh should easily come off the bone. Remove the bone, put the meat back into the stew, and stir to combine. Remove the chipotle and bay leaf and discard. Add the kale and mix well.

Serve the ragout on top of the spaghetti squash, sprinkling the parsley over the top.

Tip from Chef James: Winter squash can be hard to cut. To make it easier, put the whole squash into the oven for about 5 minutes while it's preheating. This will soften the squash and make it much easier to cut.

SEARED SALMON

Serves 4

Most people overcook fish. If you see a white substance oozing out of the fish, it is more than done. Pull it off the heat quickly. Ideally, you'd remove the fish from the pan just before you see this happen. Even better, if you're using wild, in-season salmon that was flash-frozen when caught, I highly recommend leaving it nice and rare in the middle, as this preserves the delicate omega-3 fatty acids that are such a big part of the salmon's nutritional value. Garlic Broccoli Rabe and Summer Squash (page 149) and Asparagus with Butter Mushrooms (page 147) are both great side dishes for this dish.

1 tablespoon coconut oil

2 (6-ounce) salmon fillets

Sea salt

Freshly ground black pepper

1 lemon, cut into wedges

Heat the oil in a large skillet over medium heat. Season the salmon fillets with salt and pepper, place them in the skillet, and cook for 2 to 3 minutes per side, or a bit longer for thicker fillets. Serve hot, with the lemon wedges on the side.

Breakfasts

We've all heard the saying that breakfast is the most important meal of the day. I wholeheartedly agree. A hearty, healthy breakfast will set you up for a day of feeling nourished, balanced, and satiated. The breakfast recipes we've included might take a few more minutes to prepare than a bowl of cereal, but your body will thank you. And with a little practice, you can reduce the preparation time significantly.

MUESLI

Serves 6

This breakfast is a great alternative to commercial breakfast cereals, which I don't recommend for the reasons discussed in chapter 9. Plus, it makes use of the proper preparation techniques for the oats, nuts, and seeds, soaking them overnight (in yogurt) to neutralize their antinutrients. The result is a super-speedy breakfast that maximizes the nutritional benefits of the ingredients. Once you get a handle on the basics of the recipe, try mixing up the varieties of dried fruit, nuts, and seeds.

½ cup chopped dried apricots

½ cup chopped dried apples

1 cup rolled oats (not quick-cooking oats)

¼ cup raw sunflower seeds

½ cup chopped raw pecans or almonds

½ teaspoon ground cinnamon

3 to 6 cups plain whole-milk yogurt, depending on how moist you like your muesli

Mix the apricots, apples, oats, sunflower seeds, pecans, and cinnamon together. This mixture can be stored in an airtight container for up to 1 month.

The night before serving (or even several days before), combine 1 cup of the mixture with 1 cup of yogurt (or up to 2 cups yogurt if you like it a little runny). This makes 2 to 3 servings. Cover and refrigerate overnight, then enjoy for breakfast in the morning. The soaked muesli will keep in the fridge for up to 1 week.

Tip: If fruit is in season, add some fresh fruit in the morning, as well.

EASY MORNING OATMEAL

Serves 2

This oatmeal is a good example of how to prepare grains properly, by giving them a good long soaking before cooking. You'll need to plan ahead in order to soak the oats overnight, but this step doesn't take any extra time, just a little forethought.

1 cup oats, stone-ground or rolled

2 cups filtered water

½ teaspoon ground cinnamon

⅛ teaspoon sea salt

¼ cup chopped walnuts

1 tablespoon butter

¼ cup fresh or frozen berries

1 teaspoon maple syrup

The night before, put the oats and water into a small saucepan, cover, and let stand overnight at room temperature.

In the morning, stir in the cinnamon and salt, cover, and set the pot over medium heat. Bring to a boil, then lower the heat and simmer for 10 to 15 minutes, until the oatmeal reaches the desired thickness.

Remove from the heat and stir in the walnuts and butter. If using frozen berries, add them at this point.

Divide the oatmeal equally between two bowls. If using fresh berries, sprinkle them on top at this time. Drizzle ½ teaspoon of the maple syrup over each bowl of oatmeal.

Tip: If you have very busy mornings and don't want to be in the kitchen watching over the oatmeal, try this trick: Instead of bringing the oatmeal to a boil and then turning it down, just turn the heat to its lowest setting and let the oatmeal cook slowly while you go about the rest of your morning business. It will take longer to cook, but you won't need to be in the kitchen to attend to it.

EGG-VEGGIE SCRAMBLE

Serves 2

½ cup boiling water

2 tablespoons sun-dried tomatoes

1 tablespoon and 1 teaspoon coconut oil or butter

1 cup chopped broccoli, in bite-size pieces

2 mushrooms, thinly sliced

1 small clove garlic, minced

¼ teaspoon sea salt

½ teaspoon dried oregano, or 1 teaspoon fresh

1 teaspoon water

4 eggs

2 tablespoons crumbled feta cheese or grated mozzarella cheese (optional)

Pour the boiling water over the sun-dried tomatoes and let soak for about 10 minutes, until softened. Drain and cut into thin strips.

Heat 1 tablespoon of the coconut oil in a medium skillet over medium heat. Add the broccoli, mushrooms, and garlic and sauté for 2 to 3 minutes. Stir in the sun-dried tomatoes, salt, oregano, and water. Cover and cook for 2 to 3 minutes.

Meanwhile, whisk the eggs in a small bowl. Heat the remaining coconut oil in a small skillet over medium heat, then pour in the eggs and cook, stirring occasionally, for 2 to 3 minutes or longer, depending on the desired consistency.

To serve, split the scrambled eggs between two plates and top with the sautéed vegetables. Top with the cheese and serve warm.

EGGS ON A BED OF GREENS

Serves 2

This breakfast is a standard for me. I love greens in the morning, and the poaching and steaming take very little time. With some practice, you can get the prep time for this meal down to 5 or 7 minutes, and it's such a delicious and nourishing way to start your day. Use any type of greens you like: spinach, collard greens, mustard greens, kale, Swiss chard, beet greens—whatever. One thing to note: Swiss chard, spinach, and beet greens are all high in oxalic acid (that's what makes your teeth squeaky when you eat lots of these greens), which can interfere with the absorption of some minerals. It's fine to eat these nutritious greens, but do so in moderation and alternate them with other greens.

½ teaspoon mild vinegar, such as plain white vinegar

2 very large handfuls of coarsely chopped greens (about 4 cups)

4 eggs

Grated cheese, any kind

2 tablespoons Salsa (page 142)

Freshly ground black pepper

½ avocado, sliced lengthwise

1 teaspoon freshly squeezed lime juice

Pinch of sea salt

Set up a steamer (for the greens) and bring the water to a boil. Put about 2 inches of water in a deep skillet over high heat (for poaching the eggs).

When both pans of water are boiling, turn the heat on the skillet down to medium and add the vinegar.

Put the greens in the steamer. Carefully crack the eggs into the poaching water, discarding the shells. Both the greens and the eggs should be ready within 2 to 4 minutes, depending on how runny you like your eggs. To test the eggs, poke them gently with the back of a spoon. The firmer they are, the more cooked.

To serve, divide the greens between two plates. Using a slotted spoon, carefully lift the eggs out of the poaching water one at a time, draining the water from each egg. Place 2 eggs atop each bed of greens.

Top each serving with a sprinkling of the grated cheese, half of the salsa, and pepper to taste. Arrange half of the avocado slices alongside the greens, then drizzle the lime juice over the avocado and sprinkle it with the salt.

MEXICAN EGGS
Serves 2

1 tablespoon coconut oil or butter

¼ cup diced onion

½ cup diced bell pepper, any color

Heaping ½ cup sliced zucchini, cut ¼ inch thick

¼ teaspoon sea salt

½ teaspoon paprika

4 eggs

Pinch of cayenne pepper or red pepper flakes (optional)

2 tablespoons grated Monterey Jack cheese

½ avocado, sliced lengthwise

2 tablespoons Salsa (page 142)

Heat the oil in a medium skillet over medium heat. Add the onion, bell pepper, zucchini, salt, and paprika and sauté for 2 to 3 minutes, until the onion is translucent.

Meanwhile, whisk the eggs in a small bowl. Add the eggs and cayenne to the veggie mixture and cook, stirring occasionally, for 2 to 3 minutes or longer, depending on the desired consistency.

To serve, divide the eggs between two plates and sprinkle each with half of the cheese. Top each with half of the avocado slices and half of the salsa. Serve warm.

Beverages

As discussed in chapter 10, store-bought beverages can be a big source of un-naked ingredients. Here are a few delicious and nutritious ways to make your own without all of those unnecessary and unwanted extras.

SPARKLING FLAVORED SODA

Serves 2 .

> **16 ounces (2 cups) sparkling mineral water**
>
> **½ cup freshly squeezed grapefruit juice (about 1 grapefruit)**
>
> **2 teaspoons freshly squeezed lime juice**

Combine all the ingredients, stir, and serve over ice.

Tip from Chef James: Save the grapefruit halves after juicing, and when you're cleaning your kitchen, rub them on your cutting boards and then rinse. The grapefruit will disinfect the surface naturally and leave it with a subtle citrus smell.

MINT LEMONADE

Serves 4

> **Juice of 4 lemons (about 1 cup)**
>
> **3 tablespoons raw honey or maple syrup**
>
> **¼ teaspoon grated ginger (see Tip on page 141)**
>
> **4 cups filtered water**
>
> **6 mint leaves**

Combine all the ingredients in a pitcher, whisking until thoroughly combined. Cover and refrigerate for at least 2 hours and up to 1 week.

INFUSED WATER

Serves 4

A whole new category of water has become available in stores of late: water
infused with various flavors. These drinks can be expensive, so save yourself some money and also take control of what you're drinking by making
them yourself. Try the basic version we've included here, and then experiment with your own variations. For example, you could add 4 cucumber
slices to the ingredients below. Or try lime with watermelon, cantaloupe,
or strawberries.

4 thin slices of lemon

3 thin slices of lime

4 large mint leaves

4 cups filtered water

Put the lemon and lime slices and mint leaves in a pitcher, then add the
water. Cover and refrigerate for at least 2 hours and up to 1 week. The
longer you leave it, the stronger the flavor will be.

ICED GREEN TEA

Serves 4

Why buy bottled ice tea when it's so easy to make your own? You can
adjust the sweetness and other flavors to suit your tastes. Plus, you won't
be buying a packaged product, so you'll cut down on waste (or, hopefully,
recycling).

2 green tea bags

2 thin slices of unpeeled ginger

1 slice of lemon

4 cups boiling filtered water

Up to 1 tablespoon raw honey

Put the tea bags, ginger, and lemon in a pitcher. Pour in the boiling water
and let steep for 10 to 15 minutes.

Remove the tea bags, but leave the ginger and lemon in so they keep
adding flavor to the tea. Stir in honey to taste. Let cool to room temperature, then cover and refrigerate for up to 1 week.

MANGO LASSI

Serves 2

Mango lassi is a traditional Indian drink that tastes kind of like a mango milkshake. It's quite refreshing and complements spicy foods nicely.

- 1 mango, peeled, pitted, and coarsely chopped, or 1 cup frozen mango chunks
- 1 cup filtered water
- ½ cup coconut milk
- 1 cup plain whole-milk yogurt
- ¼ teaspoon pure vanilla extract
- ½ teaspoon ground cinnamon
- Pinch of ground nutmeg

Put all the ingredients in a blender or food processor and puree until smooth. Serve immediately or store in an airtight container in the refrigerator for up to 3 days. If the lassi has been stored, stir it before serving.

Desserts

Naked treats—is there such a thing? You betcha! And they're mighty delicious. The recipes we've included are some of my favorites, and all are surprisingly easy to make. I love to bring these to potlucks to show people that eating well doesn't have to mean depriving yourself.

RAW CHOCOLATE TREATS

Makes about 12 chocolates

These rich and creamy chocolates are one of my personal favorites: imagine a chocolate treat that's so nutritionally dense you could almost consider it a supplement. They're packed with antioxidants from the chocolate and the goji berries, essential fatty acids (alpha-linolenic acid) from the walnuts, and protein from the hemp seeds. Plus, the raw honey has natural antibacterial properties. And the best part is that these chocolates are really simple to make.

This recipe uses raw cacao powder, which is not your average cocoa. It's powder from cacao beans that were cold-pressed rather than being heated to extract the cocoa liquor. This means the chocolate is truly raw—a good thing, because heat damages the delicate antioxidants in the chocolate, reducing its nutritional value significantly. When purchasing the hemp protein powder, look for a version that's made from 100 percent raw hemp seeds, ground or cold milled.

1 cup coconut oil

1 teaspoon pure vanilla extract

¼ cup hemp protein powder

¾ cup unsweetened raw cacao powder

½ cup walnuts

½ cup dried goji berries

3 tablespoons raw honey

1 teaspoon grated lime zest

1 teaspoon freshly squeezed lime juice

Combine the oil, vanilla, hemp protein, and cacao powder in a medium bowl. (If your home is a little cool, the coconut oil will be solid. If so, just turn on the oven to its lowest setting and put the coconut oil in a metal bowl in the oven. It will melt very quickly, in as little as a minute or two, and it can still be considered raw as long as it doesn't exceed a temperature of 120°F.)

Put the walnuts and goji berries in a food processor and pulse until finely ground. Transfer to the bowl with the cacao mixture and stir until thoroughly combined. Add the honey, lime zest, and lime juice and mix well.

Grease an ice cube tray with a little coconut oil. Pour the mixture into the ice cube tray, distributing it evenly, and freeze for about 20 minutes, until set.

Turn the chocolates out onto a plate. If you won't be serving them right away, cover and store in the refrigerator for up to 2 weeks.

COCONUT NUT DATE BALLS

Makes 20 balls

Like the Raw Chocolate Treats (page 174), this is dessert is raw, easy to make, and stores well in the fridge.

20 pitted dates

½ cup raw sunflower seeds

½ cup raw pecans

½ cup raw almonds

½ cup raw, unsweetened, shredded coconut

Put the dates, sunflower seeds, pecans, and almonds in a food processor and process until finely ground. Transfer the mixture to a medium bowl.

Put the coconut in a separate small bowl.

Using wet hands, form about 1½ tablespoons of the date mixture into a ball. Roll the ball in the shredded coconut until evenly covered and place on a serving plate. Continue in this way until all of the date mixture is used up, wetting your hands periodically as needed.

Freeze for about 1 hour, until set, then cover and store in the refrigerator for up to 2 weeks.

FROZEN BANANA TREATS

Serves 4

- 1 cup chopped raw pecans
- 2 tablespoons maple syrup
- ½ cup plain whole-milk yogurt
- ¼ teaspoon ground cinnamon
- 2 bananas, peeled and halved lengthwise

Preheat the oven to 375°F. Line a baking sheet with parchment paper (to help speed cleanup later).

Mix the pecans and maple syrup together, then spread the mixture on the parchment-lined baking sheet. Bake for 10 minutes, without stirring, to caramelize the nuts. (Stirring interferes with caramelizing because the sugar needs to settle. Stirring it turns it into a sticky mess.) Let the nuts cool until hardened.

Mix the yogurt and cinnamon together in a large bowl. Roll the bananas in the yogurt mixture and then the pecans, coating them evenly with the nuts.

Put the bananas on a plate or baking sheet, cover with plastic wrap, and freeze for about 3 hours, until frozen solid. Stored in the freezer, they'll keep for about 1 week.

Tip from Chef James: There are lots of possibilities for flavoring the yogurt mixture: for example, vanilla extract, raw cacao powder, or unsweetened shredded coconut. Play around with this recipe to find your favorite combination.

TOPSY-TURVY CHÈVRE FIGS
Serves 2

½ cup raw almonds or, better yet, soaked and dried almonds

4 fresh figs

1 teaspoon maple syrup

¼ teaspoon ground cinnamon

2 teaspoons chèvre

½ teaspoon balsamic vinegar

Preheat the broiler.

Put the almonds in a food processor and grind them finely. Add 2 of the figs, the maple syrup, and the cinnamon and blend to form a paste.

Cut the remaining 2 figs in half and place them, cut side down, in the bottom of 2 ramekins or small ovenproof dishes, 2 halves per ramekin. Spread 1 teaspoon of the chèvre on top of the figs in each dish. The chèvre should just cover the figs. Spread the fig paste on top of the chèvre, dividing the mixture between the two dishes. The paste should completely cover the top of the figs.

Broil for up to 8 minutes, checking every 2 minutes, until slightly browned. Using a knife, carefully scrape the sides of the ramekins. Turn the contents out, upside down, on a cutting board.

Plate the dessert with the two fig halves on top and drizzle with the balsamic vinegar. Serve warm.

MANGO COCONUT ICE POPS

Serves 10 to 12

This recipe has absolutely no added sugar and is a great replacement for commercial ice pops. They're easy and fun to make, so it's a great recipe to make with kids. And because each treat is small, the kids won't get overloaded on the fruit sugars. For molds, you can use an ice cube tray. For sticks, try wooden coffee stir sticks, cut in half. Just make sure there are no rough or sharp edges.

1 cup peeled, pitted, and coarsely chopped mango, fresh or frozen

½ cup filtered water

About ½ cup coconut milk

Put the mango and water in a blender and blend until smooth.

Pour the mixture into an ice cube tray or other molds, filling each halfway. Put a coffee stir stick into each ice pop and freeze for about 1 hour, until partially set.

Remove the ice pops from the freezer and pour the coconut milk into the molds, filling the top half of each and being careful not to overfill.

Put the ice pops back in the freezer for another 1 to 2 hours, until completely frozen through. If using an ice tray, you should be able to crack it just as you would with ice cubes. Enjoy your orange and white mini treat!

14

better than naked

I'd like to introduce you to three food-preparation techniques I've hinted at in previous chapters. I call these techniques "better than naked" because they not only preserve the nutritional value of the food, they actually enhance it. Most food preparation, including chopping, cooking, baking, juicing, and so on, actually reduces the nutritional value of the food. Cooking food damages some of the more delicate nutrients. The barbecue adds lots of flavor but that delicious charcoal flavor that makes it so distinctive comes at the cost of added carcinogens. Even something as simple as chopping diminishes the nutritional value of produce. This is just part of eating, and unless you're going to eat entirely raw foods, it's something you minimize where possible and learn to live with. Cooking minimally, chopping things right before you eat them, and eating as raw and naked as you can are some good and easy strategies for dealing with this challenge.

In some cases, you can prepare food using techniques that add to the nutritional power of the food: soaking, sprouting, and fermenting. These are powerful tools that can and do fill entire books on their own. I can't hope to delve into all the subtleties here, but I'd like to give you the basics and a short introduction to some simple ways you can prepare food to maximize its nutritional power.

Soaking

We touched on the topic of soaking in chapter 9, "Naked Grains, Beans, Nuts, and Seeds." Soaking is a useful and really easy way to prepare grains, beans, nuts, and seeds that reduces the levels and potency of antinutrients such as phytic acid. As you'll recall, grains, beans, nuts, and seeds are designed to grow another plant, not to feed our hungry bellies. In their self-preserving biological wisdom, they have nutrients in their skins that prevent premature breakdown, making them difficult to digest by inhibiting enzymatic action.

The most basic way to neutralize these antinutrients is to soak the grain, bean, nut, or seed. An easy and basic example of this is oatmeal. Instead of putting the water and oats in the pot first thing in the morning, put them in the pot the night before. In the morning, simply turn on the heat to low, and you have your oatmeal—minus most of the phytic acid. You can also soak grain in liquids other than just water. Traditional muesli is made by soaking oats, nuts, seeds, and dried fruit in either yogurt or raw milk for up to two to three days. See chapter 13 for two yummy breakfast recipes that use soaked oats.

Another common example is rice. When making a pot of rice, I'll set it to soak it in some water and leave it for at least eight hours. Before cooking the rice, I drain and rinse it. Then I add the required amount of water (or stock) for cooking, bring it to a boil, and proceed as normal.

You can (and, I would argue, should) soak any grain, bean, nut, or seed before using it. Admittedly, certain grains don't contain as many antinutrients—these are the gluten-free grains such as rice, millet, quinoa, amaranth, and buckwheat. So if you're not able to set aside the time for soaking, these are the grains to choose.

Sprouting

Sprouting takes soaking to the next level, to the point where the grain, bean, nut, or seed begins to sprout. Sprouting imparts many of the same benefits as soaking—reducing phytic acid and other enzyme inhibitors that block digestion—as well as some additional benefits. Specifically, when a grain, bean, nut, or seed has sprouted, its enzymes have "woken up," making it particularly digestible and available to your body. Essentially, when you sprout a grain, bean, nut, or seed, you trick it into thinking it's going to grow another plant, initiating that process. When you hear about "living" foods, it's referring to this enzymatic activity. Activated enzymes make digestion of the grain much easier on our bodies. Sprouting also produces or increases the vitamin content of the grain, in particular vitamin C, several of the B vitamins, and carotene (Fallon 2001).

To sprout a grain, bean, nut, or seed, all you need is a widemouthed quart-sized mason jar with some window-screen material cut to replace the insert in the lid. Fill the jar a quarter to a third full of the grain, beans, nuts, or seeds and soak the food overnight in enough filtered water to cover the food completely. In the morning, pour off the water, rinse the contents well (the mesh lid comes in handy here), drain completely, and then turn the jar upside down, setting it to rest at an angle so any remaining liquid can drain out and air can circulate. Rinse the seeds at least twice a day (if not several times). For example, try rinsing first thing in the morning and then again at night, and another time, if you think of it during the day. Depending on the size of the grain, bean, nut, or seed, it will take anywhere from one to several days for it to sprout. When it has sprouted, rinse and drain it well one last time, replace the screen insert with a solid lid, and then store in the fridge.

If the concept of sprouting is entirely new to you, pick something that's easy and common. Try sprouting some garbanzo beans (chickpeas) or mung beans in a small batch and see how you like them. Try using them in the Classic Hummus recipe on page 144.

Fermenting

Fermentation, an age-old technique used to preserve food, has a long and rich history in the human diet. From the vast variety of cultured dairy products (cheeses, yogurts, sour cream, buttermilk, kefir), to fermented fruit and vegetables (pickles, sauerkrauts), to alcohols and breads, fermentation, souring, and culturing are a fundamental part of our food preparation and preservation strategies.

When a food is fermented, microorganisms transform sugars into alcohols (grapes into wine) or lactic acids (when milk becomes cheese or cabbage becomes sauerkraut), which prevents spoilage. In the case of dairy, fermentation can increase its digestibility to the point that those who are lactose intolerant or even allergic to the proteins in milk can tolerate it. This is because most of the lactose and casein have been broken down already through the fermentation process.

As with sprouting, fermentation increases the nutritional profile of the food, adding vitamin content and beneficial bacteria that are crucial to maintaining a healthy digestive tract and immune system. The process also neutralizes any potent antinutrients present in a food. The best example of this is soy, which is loaded with antinutrients and highly indigestible until it has been fermented. Even soaking and sprouting aren't enough for soy. I've noted this already several times, but it's worth repeating—avoid all soy unless it has been fermented into tempeh, miso, tamari, or natto, a traditional Japanese dish you'll find in some Japanese restaurants.

One of my favorite foods is fermented vegetables, or "cultured veggies" as they're fondly called around our house. Traditionally prepared sauerkrauts, kimchis, pickles, and such are all the result of fermenting, or culturing, vegetables. These absolutely delicious side dishes add loads of nutritional value to the rest of your meal. Packed full of enzymes and beneficial bacteria, they are truly nutritionally dense and add such interesting flavors to your meals. As a nice bonus, they help to reduce sugar cravings and can offset the negative impact of the carcinogens in barbecued or grilled foods. This is part of the reason they're often served with meats.

You can ferment foods yourself at home, although the process differs from food to food and we don't have space here to go into that level of detail. If you'd like try fermentation at home, two excellent resources are *Nourishing Traditions* by Sally Fallon (2001) and *Wild Fermentation* by Sandor Ellix Katz (2003). You can find fermented foods at your local health-food store, but seek out those that haven't been pasteurized and are labeled "raw." Pasteurization, and heat of any kind, kills all those wonderful enzymes and beneficial bacteria that make fermented food so nutritious.

In Summary

I realize that this chapter might seem to take naked foods to a whole new level. I include it not to overwhelm you and not really as a starting point. These concepts and techniques are fun to play with once you've already shifted much of your diet over to a naked one. This is the next level, a starting point for some truly traditional, incredibly nourishing food preparation techniques. If you're new to the idea of naked foods, bookmark this chapter and come back to it later. If you're a naked-foods pro, try some of these techniques and check out some of the resources I've included on my website (www.eatnakednow.com).

15

when *not* to eat naked

I have a confession to make. Sometimes I don't eat naked. I know. It's shocking, but it's true. In fact, sometimes I eat wildly un-naked foods. And you know what? When I do, I love every minute of it.

So here's the chapter where I advise you to take all of this with a grain of salt. Of course I think it's critically important that we be mindful of what we put in our mouths and how we nourish our bodies. Of course I am deeply concerned about the health crisis that sits in front of us, and I am clearly of the mind that our food plays an enormous and pivotal role in this situation. I certainly would never advocate a diet of mostly processed and un-naked foods. And yet, there is a time and place for such things.

As any of my clients will tell you, I am a big believer in keeping it real. I don't believe in deprivation, and I don't believe in strict diets that give you no room to bend the rules. In fact, I think inflexibility isn't much healthier than not giving a rat's ass about what you put in your mouth. Both are extremes and, in my mind, terribly out of balance.

There's a concept called *orthorexia* that describes someone who obsesses and fixates upon eating healthy, pure food. While in some cases this is necessary for very specific and real health reasons—as in the case of an allergy—this obsession can take on its own life and drive you (and those around you) a little mad.

My intention with this book and the information I've shared with you is certainly not to drive you to orthorexia. I can feel the raised eyebrows of those who have known me over the years, and yes, I can lean to the obsessive side of things at times myself. That's exactly why I've included this chapter. It's as much a reminder for me as it is for you. It's okay to bend the rules. In fact, it's important to bend the rules every once in a while.

Making It Stick Means Keeping It Real

I think the key to making real, lasting, sustainable changes in our lives is all about making them truly realistic. The problem I see with the all-or-nothing tendency is that it sets us up for failure from the get-go. There's a perfectionist streak running through our culture. I see it all the time with myself and with my clients. It manifests as a commitment to making a change, followed by a sincere effort at rigidly doing it "right." Then something invariably happens (you know, life), and we fall off the wagon—at which point we throw our hands despairingly into the air and give up.

But what if we built a little off-wagon time into the package? What if part of the whole thing was an understanding up front that there are times we want to indulge in "guilty" pleasures? What if that wasn't only okay, but an acknowledged, accepted, dare I say celebrated part of the process?

Fundamentally, it's not about whether you indulged in a double-fudge sundae with extra whipping cream. It's about what you're doing most of the time, day in, day out. Here are the guidelines I use to keep it real.

My 80:20 Rule

I use a variation of the 80:20 rule applied to food. If 80 percent of my food is naked—fresh, whole, organic, homemade—then for the other 20 percent, I don't worry about it. What's important is what you're feeding yourself the bulk of the time. That's where to focus your energy. If there's a favorite food you absolutely adore and it's not naked, oh well. Don't eat it every day, but have it occasionally as a treat.

I'm going to share a personal tidbit here that's wildly ironic and certainly not something I thought would ever go into print. You have now been on this journey with me and understand how passionate I am about real, whole, healthy, naked foods. They make my heart sing and my body thrive. And yet, my most basic comfort food is one of the most un-naked foods there is: boxed macaroni and cheese. Not the hearty, homemade variety my Gramma used to make. I'm talking about the fluorescent orange powdered cheese with white noodles. The only thing remotely nutritious about it is the milk and butter I add to the sauce.

There were times as I was writing this book that I struggled to finish chapters or to meet a deadline. I was stretching way out of my comfort zone, and as a result, I was craving deep comfort—something I, like many others, find in food. And the comfort food I was craving was mac and cheese out of a box.

I could have done many different things with these cravings. I could have simply denied them and plowed forward, making it a matter of will-power (for the record, I don't believe in willpower, but that's a topic for another book). I could have indulged my cravings mindlessly. I could have beaten myself up for having them despite "knowing better." But I didn't do any of these things. I laughed about the irony and then used the craving as incentive. I rewarded myself for a chapter completed with a box of the stuff, eaten straight out of the pot with a wooden spoon in front of some bad TV crime show with a glass of wine. And I savored every little mouthful of it.

Which brings me to my next point...

Indulge and Enjoy!

Now here's the only rule I will ever strictly enforce with myself and with others. If you are going to have that treat, if you're going to indulge in some guilty pleasure, then the absolute most important thing is that you truly, fully enjoy it. Eating something you think you shouldn't and beating yourself up about it the whole time—something that I see people do every single day—is far, far more damaging to your body than eating that very same food and delighting in it.

How you feel when you eat your dinner has about as much impact on how your body uses that food as what it is you're eating. In chapter 11, "Transitioning to a Naked Diet," we looked at the importance of being in a relaxed state when eating so that your digestion is maximized. Stress compromises digestion, and guilt is most definitely stress inducing.

I was once asked at a workshop about what on earth I order from a restaurant menu. My response: "Whatever I want, and I enjoy it." And that's exactly what I do. I check in with myself and see what I feel like eating. I don't overthink it, and I don't analyze the nutritional pros and cons of the various options. I just eat what I feel like eating. And, most importantly, I enjoy every little mouthful of it.

So, when I do eat the mac and cheese, or I pick something off a menu that's clearly not naked, I eat it with delight, not guilt. And I encourage you to do the same.

In Summary

Eating naked is something to strive for, to move toward step-by-step, and to do as much of the time as you can. It's how your body will thrive and your waistline will shrink. And, for this to be a sustainable lifestyle for you, it's important to build in some wiggle room. The more naked you eat, the fewer of these guilty pleasures you will crave as your body resets and your standards rise. It's your journey. Enjoy it.

References

American Heart Association. 2010. Sodium (salt or sodium chloride). www.american heart.org/print_presenter.jhtml?identifier=4708. Accessed December 9, 2010.

Angell, S. 2010. Emerging opportunities for monitoring the nutritional content of processed foods. *American Journal of Clinical Nutrition* 91(2):298–299.

Aoki, Y. 2001. Polychlorinated biphenyls, polychlorinated dibenzo-p-dioxins, and polychlorinated dibenzofurans as endocrine disrupters—what we have learned from Yusho disease. *Environmental Research* 86(1):2–11.

Basciano, H., L. Federico, and K. Adeli. 2005. Fructose, insulin resistance, and metabolic dyslipidemia. *Nutrition and Metabolism* 2(1):5.

Batmanghelidj, F. 1997. *Your Body's Many Cries for Water.* Vienna, VA: Global Health Solutions.

Beck-Nielsen, H., O. Pedersen, and N. S. Sørensen. 1978. Effects of diet on the cellular insulin binding and the insulin sensitivity in young healthy subjects. *Diabetologia* 15(4):289–296.

Belury, M. A. 2002. Inhibition of carcinogenesis by conjugated linoleic acid: Potential mechanisms of action. *Journal of Nutrition* 132(10):2995–2998.

Blankson, H., J. A. Stakkestad, H. Fagertun, E. Thom, J. Wadstein, and O. Gudmundsen. 2000. Conjugated linoleic acid reduces body fat mass in overweight and obese humans. *Journal of Nutrition* 130(12):2943–2948.

Callaway, T. R., R. O. Elder, J. E. Keen, R. C. Anderson, and D. J. Nisbet. 2003. Forage feeding to reduce preharvest *Escherichia coli* populations in cattle, a review. *Journal of Dairy Science* 86(3):852–860.

Celiac Disease Center at Columbia University Medical Center. No date. Frequently asked questions. www.celiacdiseasecenter.columbia.edu/A_Patients/A02-FAQ.htm. Accessed December 9, 2010.

Chajès, V., A. C. Thiébaut, M. Rotival, E. Gauthier, V. Maillard, M. C. Boutron-Ruault, V. Joulin, G. M. Lenoir, and F. Clavel-Chapelon. 2008. Association between serum trans-monounsaturated fatty acids and breast cancer risk in the E3N-EPIC Study. *American Journal of Epidemiology* 167(11):1312–1320.

Chavarro, J. E., J. W. Rich-Edwards, B. A. Rosner, and W. C. Willett. 2007. Dietary fatty acid intakes and the risk of ovulatory infertility. *American Journal of Clinical Nutrition* 85(1):231–237.

Christensen, L. 1991. The role of caffeine and sugar in depression. *Nutrition Report* 9(3):17–24.

Colantuoni, C., P. Rada, J. McCarthy, C. Patten, N. Avena, A. Chadeayne, and B. G. Hoebel. 2002. Evidence that intermittent, excessive sugar intake causes endogenous opioid dependence. *Obesity Research* 10(6):478–488.

Cornée, J., D. Pobel, E. Riboli, M. Guyader, and B. Hémon. 1995. A case-control study of gastric cancer and nutritional factors in Marseille, France. *European Journal of Epidemiology* 11(1):55–65.

Damsgaard, C. T., L. Lauritzen, T. M. Kjær, P. M. Holm, M. B. Fruekilde, K. F. Michaelsen, and H. Frøkiær. 2007. Fish oil supplementation modulates immune function in healthy infants. *Journal of Nutrition* 137(4):1031–1036.

Daniel, K. T. 2005. *The Whole Soy Story: The Dark Side of America's Favorite Health Food.* Washington, DC: New Trends Publishing.

David, M. 2005. *The Slow Down Diet: Eating for Pleasure, Energy, and Weight Loss.* Rochester, VT: Healing Arts Press.

De Deckere, E. A. 1999. Possible beneficial effect of fish and fish n-3 polyunsaturated fatty acids in breast and colorectal cancer. *European Journal of Cancer Prevention* 8(3):213–221.

De Stefani, E., H. D. Pellegrini, M. Mendilaharsu, A. Ronco, and J. C. Carzoglio. 1998. Dietary sugar and lung cancer: A case-control study in Uruguay. *Nutrition and Cancer* 31(2):132–137.

Dhiman, T. R., G. R. Anand, L. D. Satter, and M. W. Pariza. 1999. Conjugated linoleic acid content of milk from cows fed different diets. *Journal of Dairy Science* 82(10):2146–2156.

Enig, M. G. 2000. *Know Your Fats: The Complete Primer for Understanding the Nutrition of Fats, Oils, and Cholesterol.* Silver Spring, MD: Bethesda Press.

Enig, M. G., and S. Fallon. 2006. *Eat Fat, Lose Fat: The Healthy Alternative to Trans Fat.* New York: Plume.

Environmental Protection Agency. 2009. *Chemicals Evaluated for Carcinogenic Potential.* Washington, DC: EPA, Science Information Management Branch, Health Effects Division, Office of Pesticide Programs.

Environmental Working Group. 2010. *2010 Shopper's Guide to Pesticides.* Washington, DC: Environmental Working Group.

Fallon, S., with M. G. Enig. 2001. *Nourishing Traditions: The Cookbook That Challenges Politically Correct Nutrition and the Diet Dictocrats.* Washington, DC: New Trends Publishing.

Ferreira, M., M. Caetano, P. Antunes, J. Costa, O. Gil, N. Bandarra, P. Pousão-Ferreira, C. Vale, and M. A. Reis-Henriques. 2010. Assessment of contaminants and biomarkers of exposure in wild and farmed seabass. *Ecotoxicology and Environmental Safety* 73(4):579–588.

Flower, K. B., J. A. Hoppin, C. F. Lynch, A. Blair, C. Knott, D. L. Shore, and D. P. Sandler. 2004. Cancer risk and parental pesticide application in children of agricultural health study participants. *Environmental Health Perspectives* 112(5):631–635.

Food and Agriculture Organization of the United Nations. 2005. *Review of the State of World Marine Fishery Resources*. Rome, Italy: FAO.

Foran, J. A., D. O. Carpenter, M. C. Hamilton, B. A. Knuth, and S. J. Schwager. 2005. Risk-based consumption advice for farmed Atlantic and wild Pacific salmon contaminated with dioxins and dioxin-like compounds. *Environmental Health Perspectives* 113(5):552–556.

Fowler, S. P., K. Williams, R. G. Resendez, K. J. Hunt, H. P. Hazuda, and M. P. Stern. 2008. Fueling the obesity epidemic? Artificially sweetened beverage use and long-term weight gain. *Obesity* 16(8):1894–1900.

Goldburg, R. J., M. S. Elliott, and R. L. Naylor. 2001. *Marine Aquaculture in the United States: Environmental Impacts and Policy Options*. Arlington, VA: Pew Oceans Commission.

Grant, E. C., 1979. Food allergies and migraines. *Lancet* 313(8123):966–969.

Hu, F. B., M. J. Stampfer, E. B. Rimm, J. E. Manson, A. Ascherio, G. A. Colditz, B. A. Rosner, D. Spiegelman, F. E. Speizer, F. M. Sacks, C. H. Hennekens, and W. C. Willett. 1999. A prospective study of egg consumption and risk of cardiovascular disease in men and women. *Journal of the American Medical Association* 281(15):1387–1394.

Institute of Medicine. 2002. *Dietary Reference Intakes for Energy, Carbohydrate, Fiber, Fat, Fatty Acids, Cholesterol, Protein, and Amino Acids*. Washington, DC: National Academies Press.

Johnson, R. J., and T. Gower. 2008. *The Sugar Fix: The High-Fructose Fallout That Is Making You Sick and Fat*. New York: Rodale Press.

Katz, S. E. 2003. *Wild Fermentation: The Flavor, Nutrition, and Craft of Live-Culture Foods*. White River Junction, VT: Chelsea Green Publishing Company.

Kavanagh, K., K. L. Jones, J. Sawyer, K. Kelley, J. J. Carr, J. D. Wagner, and L. L. Rudel. 2007. Trans fat diet induces abdominal obesity and changes in insulin sensitivity in monkeys. *Obesity (Silver Spring)* 15(7):1675–1684.

Keith, L. 2009. *The Vegetarian Myth: Food, Justice, and Sustainability*. Oakland, CA: Flashpoint Press.

Kelsay J. L., K. M. Behall, J. M. Holden, and E. S. Prather. 1974. Diets high in glucose or sucrose and young women. *American Journal of Clinical Nutrition* 27(9):926–936.

Kinsella, J. E. 1987. Effects of polyunsaturated fatty acids on factors related to cardiovascular disease. *American Journal of Cardiology* 60(12):23G–32G.

Koehler, S. M., and A. Glaros. 1988. The effect of aspartame on migraine headache. *Headache: Journal of Head and Face Pain* 28(1):10–14.

Kritchevsky, S. B., and D. Kritchevsky. 2000. Egg consumption and coronary heart disease: An epidemiologic overview. *Journal of the American College of Nutrition* 19(5):549S–555S.

Lappé, A. 2009. The climate crisis at the end of our fork. In *Food, Inc: A Participant's Guide*, edited by Karl Weber, 105–118. New York: Participant Media.

LaSalle, T. J., and P. Hepperly. 2008. *Regenerative Organic Farming: A Solution to Global Warming*. Kutztown, PA: Rodale Institute.

Liu, S., W. C. Willett, M. J. Stampfer, F. B. Hu, M. Franz, L. Sampson, C. H. Hennekens, and J. E. Manson. 2000. A prospective study of dietary glycemic load, carbohydrate intake, and risk of coronary heart disease in U.S. women. *American Journal of Clinical Nutrition* 71(6):1455–1461.

Mateljan, G. 2007. *The World's Healthiest Foods*. Seattle, WA: George Mateljan Foundation Publishing.

Mayo Clinic Staff. 2009. Food allergies: Watch food labels for these top 8 allergens. www.mayoclinic.com/health/food-allergies/aa00057. Accessed December 11, 2010.

McAfee, M. 2010. The fifteen things that pasteurization kills. *Wise Traditions in Food, Farming, and the Healing Arts* 11(2):82–86.

McKenney, J. M., and D. Sica. 2007. Prescription omega-3 fatty acids for the treatment of hypertriglyceridemia. *American Journal of Health-System Pharmacists* 64(6):595–605.

Mensink, R. P., and M. B. Katan. 1990. Effect of dietary trans fatty acids on high-density and low-density lipoprotein cholesterol levels in healthy subjects. *New England Journal of Medicine* 323(7):439–445.

Mercola, J., and K. D. Pearsall. 2000. *Sweet Deception*. Nashville, TN: Thomas Nelson.

Mischoulon, D., G. I. Papakostas, C. M. Dording, A. H. Farabaugh, S. B. Sonawalla, A. M. Agoston, J. Smith, E. C. Beaumont, L. E. Dahan, J. E. Alpert, A. A. Nierenberg, and M. Fava. 2009. A double-blind, randomized controlled trial of ethyl-eicosapentaenoate for major depressive disorder. *Journal of Clinical Psychiatry* 70(12):1636–1644.

Mitchell, A. E., Y. J. Hong, E. Koh, D. M. Barrett, D. E. Bryant, R. F. Denison, and S. Kaffka. 2007. Ten-year comparison of the influence of organic and conventional crop-management practices on the content of flavonoids in tomatoes. *Journal of Agricultural and Food Chemistry* 55(15):6154–6159.

Moerman, C. J., H. B. Bueno de Mesquita, and S. Runia. 1993. Dietary sugar intake in the aetiology of biliary tract cancer. *International Journal of Epidemiology* 22(2):207–214.

Muskiet, F. A., M. R. Fokkema, A. Schaafsma, E. R. Boersma, and M. A. Crawford. 2004. Is docosahexaenoic acid (DHA) essential? Lessons from DHA status regulation, our ancient diet, epidemiology and randomized controlled trials. *Journal of Nutrition* 134(1):183–186.

Nagel, R 2010. Living with phytic acid: Preparing grains, nuts, seeds, and beans for maximum nutrition. *Wise Traditions in Food, Farming, and the Healing Arts* 11(1):28–39.

Nestle, M. 2006. *What to Eat*. New York: North Point Press.

Ogden, C. L., and M. D. Carroll. 2010. Prevalence of overweight, obesity, and extreme obesity among adults: United States, trends 1976–1980 through 2007–2008. Atlanta, GA: Center for Disease Control, National Center for Health Statistics.

Olshansky, S. J., D. J. Passaro, R. C. Hershow, J. Layden, B. A. Carnes, J. Brody, L. Hayflick, R. N. Butler, D. B. Allison, and D. S. Ludwig. 2005. A potential decline in life expectancy in the United States in the 21st century. *New England Journal of Medicine* 352(11):1138–1145.

Parks, E. J., L. E. Skokan, M. T. Timlin, and C. S. Dingfelder. 2008. Dietary sugars stimulate fatty acid synthesis in adults. *Journal of Nutrition* 138(6):1039–1046.

Pitchford, P. 2002. *Healing with Whole Foods: Asian Traditions and Modern Wisdom.* Berkeley, CA: North Atlantic Books.

Planck, N. 2006. *Real Food: What to Eat and Why.* New York: Bloomsbury Press.

Pollan, M. 2009. *In Defense of Food: An Eater's Manifesto.* New York: Penguin.

Ravnskov, U. 1998. The questionable role of saturated and polyunsaturated fatty acids in cardiovascular disease. *Journal of Clinical Epidemiology* 51(6):443–460.

Reaven, P., S. Parthasarathy, B. J. Grasse, E. Miller, D. Steinberg, and J. L. Witztum. 1991. Feasibility of using an oleate-rich diet to reduce the susceptibility of low-density lipoprotein to oxidative modification in humans. *American Journal of Clinical Nutrition* 54(4):701–761.

Reiser, S. 1985. Effect of dietary sugars on metabolic risk factors associated with heart disease. *Nutrition and Health* 3(4):203–216.

Reiser, S., J. Hallfrisch, M. Fields, A. Powell, W. Mertz, E. S. Prather, and J. J. Canary. 1986. Effects of sugars on indices of glucose tolerance in humans. *American Journal of Clinical Nutrition* 43(1):151–159.

Robbins, J. 1987. *Diet for a New America.* Novato, CA: New World Library.

Rosenthal, J. 2008. *Integrative Nutrition: Feed Your Hunger for Health and Happiness.* New York: Integrative Nutrition Publishing.

Sanchez, A., J. L. Reeser, H. S. Lau, P. Y. Yahiku, R. E. Willard, P. J. McMillan, S. Y. Cho, A. R. Magie, and U. D. Register. 1973. Role of sugars in human neutrophilic phagocytosis. *American Journal of Clinical Nutrition* 26(11):1180–1184.

Sanda, B. 2004. The double danger of high-fructose corn syrup. *Wise Traditions in Food, Farming, and the Healing Arts* 4(4):16–23.

Schmid, R. 2003. *The Untold Story of Milk: Green Pastures, Contented Cows, and Raw Dairy Foods.* Washington, DC: New Trends Publishing.

Smith, G. C., J. B. Morgan, J. N. Sofos, and J. D. Tatum. 1996. Dietary supplementation of vitamin E to cattle to improve shelf life and case life of beef for domestic and international markets. *Animal Feed Science and Technology* 59(1):207–214.

Squire, R. A. 1985. Histopathological evaluation of rat urinary bladders from the IRDC two-generation bioassay of sodium saccharin. *Food and Chemical Toxicology* 23(4–5):491–497.

Steinfeld, H., P. Gerber, T. Wassenaar, V. Castel, M. Rosales, and C. De Haan. 2006. *Livestock's Long Shadow: Environmental Issues and Options.* Rome, Italy: Food and Agriculture Organization of the United Nations.

Sundram, K, T. Karupaiah, and K. C. Hayes. 2007. Stearic acid–rich interesterified fat and trans-rich fat raise the LDL/HDL ratio and plasma glucose relative to palm olein in humans. *Nutrition and Metabolism* 4:3.

Swithers, S. E., and T. L. Davidson. 2008. A role for sweet taste: Calorie predictive relations in energy regulation by rats. *Behavioral Neuroscience* 122(1):161–173.

Taylor, J. M., M. A. Weinberger, and L. Friedman. 1980. Chronic toxicity and carcinogenicity to the urinary bladder of sodium saccharin in the in utero–exposed rat. *Toxicology and Applied Pharmacology* 54(1):57–75.

Thomas, B. J., R. J. Jarrett, H. Keen, and H. J. Ruskin. 1982. Relation of habitual diet to fasting plasma insulin concentration and the insulin response to oral glucose. *Human Nutrition. Clinical Nutrition* 36C(1):49–56.

TransFair USA. No date. About fair trade. www.transfairusa.org/content/ certification. Accessed December 11, 2010.

U.S. Department of Agriculture. 2006. National organic program: Access to pasture (livestock). *Federal Register* 75(31):7154–7195. Available at www.ams. usda.gov/AMSv1.0/getfile?dDocName=STELPRDC5082838&acct=noprulem aking. Accessed December 9, 2010.

U.S. Department of Agriculture. 2010. Fact sheets: Food labeling: Meat and poultry labeling terms. Washington, DC: USDA, Food Safety and Inspection Service. Available at www.fsis.usda.gov/factsheets/Meat_&_Poultry_Labeling_ Terms/index.asp. Accessed December 9, 2010.

U.S. Geological Survey. 1999. *U.S. Geological Survey Circular 1225: The Quality of Our Nation's Waters—Nutrients and Pesticides.* Reston, VA: U.S. Geological Survey.

Vallejo, F., F. A. Tomas-Barberan, and C. Garcia-Viguera. 2003. Phenolic compound contents in edible parts of broccoli inflorescences after domestic cooking. *Journal of the Science of Food and Agriculture* 83(14):1511–1516.

Van Boekel, M. A. 1991. The role of glycation in aging and diabetes mellitus. *Molecular Biology Report* 15(2):57–64.

Vos, M. B., J. E. Kimmons, C. Gillespie, J. Welsh, and H. M. Blanck. 2008. Dietary fructose consumption among U.S. children and adults: The third national health and nutrition examination survey. *Medscape Journal of Medicine* 10(7):160.

Weston A. Price Foundation. 2000. *Principles of Healthy Diets.* Washington, DC: Weston A. Price Foundation.

Willet, W. C., M. J. Stampfer, J. E. Manson, G. A. Colditz, F. E. Speizer, B. A. Rosner, L. A. Sampson, and C. H. Hennekens. 1993. Intake of trans fatty acids and risk of coronary heart disease among women. *Lancet* 341(8845):581–585.

World Health Organization. 2002. Global and regional food consumption patterns and trends. In *Report of the Joint WHO/FAO Expert Consultation on Diet, Nutrition, and the Prevention of Chronic Diseases*, Geneva, Switzerland, January 28–February 1.

Worthington, V. 2001. Nutritional quality of organic versus conventional fruits, vegetables, and grains. *Journal of Alternative and Complementary Medicine* 7(2):161–173.

Xu, J., K. D. Kochanek, S. L. Murphy, and B. Tejada-Vera. 2010. Deaths: Final data for 2007. *National Vital Statistics Reports* 58(19).

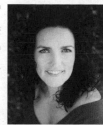

Jasmine Lord

Margaret Floyd is a nutritional therapy practitioner, certified holistic health counselor, certified healing foods specialist, and certified member of the American Association of Drugless Practitioners. She lives in Los Angeles, CA, where she has a thriving practice, serving clients around the world. Visit the author online at www.eatnakednow.com.

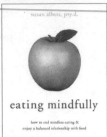
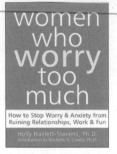
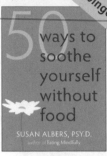
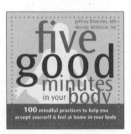
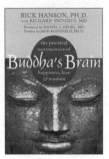
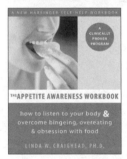